CRYSTALS

The Definitive Holistic Guide for Learning How Stones

(The Beginner's Guide to Discover the Power and Positive Energy)

Jean McAllister

Published by Harry Barnes

Jean McAllister

All Rights Reserved

Crystals: The Definitive Holistic Guide for Learning How Stones (The Beginner's Guide to Discover the Power and Positive Energy)

ISBN 978-1-7751430-5-5

All rights reserved. No part of this guide may be reproduced in any form without permission in writing from the publisher except in the case of brief quotations embodied in critical articles or reviews.

Legal & Disclaimer

The information contained in this book is not designed to replace or take the place of any form of medicine or professional medical advice. The information in this book has been provided for educational and entertainment purposes only.

The information contained in this book has been compiled from sources deemed reliable, and it is accurate to the best of the Author's knowledge; however, the Author cannot guarantee its accuracy and validity and cannot be held liable for any errors or omissions. Changes are periodically made to this book. You must consult your doctor or get professional medical advice before using any of the suggested remedies, techniques, or information in this book.

Upon using the information contained in this book, you agree to hold harmless the Author from and against any damages, costs, and expenses, including any legal fees potentially resulting from the application of any of the information provided by this guide. This disclaimer applies to any damages or injury caused by the use and application, whether directly or indirectly, of any advice or information presented, whether for breach of contract, tort, negligence, personal injury, criminal intent, or under any other cause of action.

You agree to accept all risks of using the information presented inside this book. You need to consult a professional medical practitioner in order to ensure you are both able and healthy enough to participate in this program.

Table of Contents

INTRODUCTION 1

CHAPTER 1: CRYSTAL ROOTS & FOUNDATIONS 10

CHAPTER 2: HOW CRYSTALS WORK 32

CHAPTER 3: CRYSTAL THERAPISTS 36

CHAPTER 4: HOW TO PREPARE FOR NATURAL AND MANMADE DISASTERS 49

CHAPTER 5: HOW CRYSTAL HEALING WORKS 54

CHAPTER 6: EVERYDAY USES FOR HEALING CRYSTALS 57

CHAPTER 7: STONES AND THEIR HEALING PROPERTIES ... 88

CHAPTER 8: YOUR OWN COLLECTION 121

CHAPTER 9: DIAMOND 153

CHAPTER 6: IMPORTANT CRYSTALS, THEIR USES, AND THEIR HEALING POWERS 166

CONCLUSION 203

Introduction

Crystals have been around for millions of years and have played an important role in human culture since prehistoric times. With their dazzling colors and unusual shapes and textures, they must have looked like something out of this world and it's hardly surprising they were used for magic, religious ceremonies and initiations.

How early man managed to figure out their healing properties we'll never know, but a lot of what we know about the use of crystal in healing and magic comes from ancient Egypt. They may not have been the first ones to discover these properties but were the first ones to record them for posterity.

Since 500,000 BC, when the oldest clear quartz tools were discovered in a cave near Beijing, crystals have been part of our everyday life, in one way or another. Although our knowledge about crystals has grown and they've become an indispensable component of high-tech programs, our fascination with their magical and healing powers has not diminished. On the contrary.

Objects of great beauty, but also powerful healing tools whose impact on human body and psyche we are only beginning to understand, crystals continue to fascinate us. It was only relatively recently we realized that healing takes place not only on a physical but also on emotional and spiritual levels as well.

There are now also chakrubs: mineral sex toys that literally work from the inside. An egg-shaped quartz, for example, is supposed to clean and unleash energy after insertion into the vagina. Some women report that the energy flow initially overwhelmed them and that doesn't mean orgasm, not satisfaction, but general satisfaction.

With a correct crystal therapy, different stones are placed on different parts of the body. Moonstone can intensify feelings, amethyst has a calming effect. Citrine is also called the stone of success and is the yellow colored variation of quartz; it brings luck and deepens optimism. The green aventurine keeps the energy of wealth and new opportunities. Rose quartz - one of the most popular stones - spreads positive energy, in love, as well as in the job. Bosses place it on the desk to let the forces flow through the offices. Katy Perry once said that with a rose quartz in her pocket, she doesn't stay single for long.

If you want to experience the effect of crystals more visually, you should think about crystal therapy as a beauty treatment, which is also popular right now. If you drive a rose quartz over your skin, it should make you look younger - the crystal stimulates blood circulation and the lymphatic system and has a detoxifying, visibly decongestant effect. In turn, hematite is said to give young skin new energy. Amethyst soothes the skin so that redness and pimples disappear. Hollywood stars like Jennifer Aniston and Emma Stone swear by crystals for beauty, which are regularly treated by the New York beautician Georgia Alice. If you don't believe in spirituality, you may believe in the latest beauty hype.

The magic of crystals lies in their ability to pick up vibrations from their environment, and in case of negative energy, to transform it into something positive and good. In the case of positive energy, they are able to amplify it for the benefit of all those who happen to find themselves in such an environment.

Ancient knowledge and practice we so easily renounced as legends and old wives' tales, is something we are now struggling to restore and bring back to life. Unfortunately, much of it has been irretrievably lost, but as more and more people struggle to cope with the increasing stress and uncertainty of the modern world, the need for ancient wisdom is more important than ever.

The ancient Greeks asked the big questions about what it means to live a good life, and some of their theories on ethics and happiness have been backed by modern science. Let's hope the shift in human consciousness, which is underway, will help restore the place crystals once held in human culture.

How Crystals Work

By now, you can probably begin to realize exactly how important it is to balance your chakras. While researchers are still studying links between the spiritual, emotional, mental, and physical realms, the chakra system is backed by thousands of years of practice. Innumerable people across decades and all parts of the world have found that taking proper care to maintain their chakras is an effective way to boost mental and physical health and to combat serious issues.

In fact, many of the potential issues listed above that can result from imbalanced chakras seem quite frightening - you probably didn't know that diseases found in major organs could be affected by something like your energy field. Yet, it makes sense - after all, each of us is made up of energy, and the way in which our energy reacts with that of our surroundings naturally has an effect on us. Of course, sometimes this effect can be positive, but in many cases, the toxins and negative energy sources we're exposed to have a detrimental effect on us.

That's why crystals are so important. Despite efforts to eat clean, reduce your carbon footprint, or exercise regularly, your chakras still need an extra boost to be perfectly regulated. Healing crystals hold the key to unlocking unlimited wellness potential within your mind and body.

It seems crazy, probably, to anyone who isn't familiar with the concept. How could a rock possibly have any sort of healing processes? We'll explain.

As we mentioned above, the most important aspect of balancing your chakras is ensuring the fact that their vibratory frequencies are resonating at their ideal levels. An irregularity can occur from a disturbance, which causes the vibratory pattern to be thrown off. Consequently, we feel out of sorts, either in mental or physical capacity, or both. Healing crystals, then, have the capacity to regulate these patterns and restore harmony within our chakras.

To explain it simply, crystals, like all other aspects of our world, have their own distinct vibratory patterns. Yet, healing crystals emit some of the purest resonances, thanks to their innate, balanced structure. The vibrations they offer our chakras act as tuning forks, bringing our energy field back to the level at which it vibrates most efficiently, thereby restoring health and harmony. Yet, you must allow yourself to be mentally, physically, and spiritually receptive to these restorations, which can be an issue for some nonbelievers.

To anyone who discredits the value of healing crystals, it's important to understand that there is, in fact, a scientific facet to this practice. Think of it this way: it's a known fact that despite the classifications of gasses, liquids, and solids, nothing is ever truly wholly "solid;" rather, anything that's solid is made up of a series of moving atoms, in addition to molecules and minerals. Thus, the atoms that are moving among us have an energy about them.

People, therefore, are complex beings, made up of energy fields that embody nature's balance and organizational properties. Just as our chakra patterns are unique, so, too, is each crystal. The pattern at which each stone resonates corresponds best with specific chakras. To heal ourselves holistically, we can choose certain crystals to best harmonize the chakras among us that may have experienced an imbalance. Each crystal is an active participant in nature with a valuable purpose.

Chapter 1: Crystal Roots & Foundations

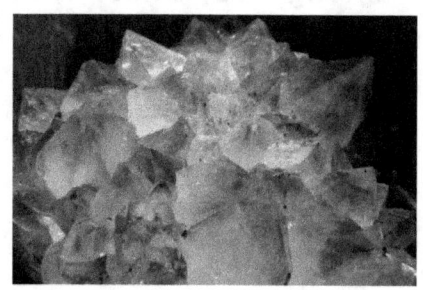

Crystal Roots & Origins

Crystals, otherwise known as **gemstones** or **rare gems**, have been around for thousands of years. They have been around since the start of time, being formed directly from the earth and mother earth's energies. Crystals begin their life as a microcrystalline collective (again, formed directly from the earth). The microcrystal structures grow to create the larger crystals we see today. Larger crystals not formed from microcrystalline layers are formed from hot lava on the earth's surface, also known as pegmatite. Some crystal clusters, or intergrown crystals, are more specifically formed from this type of formation. Amethyst geodes, for example, are a prime example. Crystals are influenced from the natural world and elemental energies just as we are. Crystals are essentially formed from 'stresses' in the earth's movement, stresses which occur when layers of rock slide over one another, and usually in a repetitive or continuous movement from gravitational forces in the earth. In this sense, crystals are highly influenced and created from the sun, moon, and other planets which- as we explore later- do not have a solely physical effect. The effect of the planets and astrological happenings above is what creates the **metaphysical** and healing properties we receive from the crystal queen/kingdom.

It is interesting to note that crystals are usually referred to as the crystal **kingdom**. But what about the crystal **queendom**?

That is the beauty with this book and why it is unique (truly!) this book offers a balanced, whole and integrated approach and takes into consideration the feminine energies that construct and shape life on earth, and we humans- something that can often go overlooked in a masculine-steered society! One significant perspective you will grow to understand and embody throughout these chapters is how crystals embody unique and specific feminine **and** masculine energies. Just like us humans and other natural entities such as flower essences, herbs, and plants; crystals have their own physiology of characteristics. Although it is not widely taught or even considered by many as a truth, the fact that we refer to gemstones (and many other entities in nature such as animals) as 'kingdoms,' not queendoms, inherently suggests some sort of imbalance and possibly even suppression. It is known that the concept of crystals and their healing powers aren't taught widely-they are not included as part of the national curriculum and many people don't find out about crystals and their beneficial properties until they begin their own journey of discovery. So, as we live in a predominantly patriarchal society (as opposed to matriarchal), we can imply that the exclusion of crystals and suppression of certain wisdom and esoteric knowledge is closely linked to deeply ingrained beliefs, societal conditionings, and bias choices of language. The crystal world, whether kingdom or queendom links strongly with our earth, the **Great Mother**. And the earth is primarily a feminine principle, just as the sun is masculine. It is important to make this distinction and bring this into awareness, there is great insight to be gained through our fundamental choice of language, reasoning, and logic.

Learning about crystals and seeking to embody their wisdom will allow you to connect with the subtle energy and subsequent healing benefits. You will become open to new and evolved ways of perceiving things, further opening your mind and heart to the beauty and unity of the natural world. Crystals are conscious, they continuously interact with other living entities including our own auras, or electromagnetic energy fields. The consciousness of crystals can become our consciousness.

Astrological Influences

Astrological transits and planets in our orbit influence every aspect of life on earth, including our own personalities, desires, likes and dislikes, passions, strengths and weaknesses, and the vibrational qualities of crystals and rare gems. We ourselves are born with a unique set of planetary positions, including sun sign, moon sign, rising/ascendant, and all of the other planets. The metaphysical and healing properties of crystals are affected and enhanced by astrological influences up above; every living entity has an aura, and electromagnetic energy field that interacts with the electromagnetic fields of others. In this sense, we are all interconnected (picture a hologram!). The planets influence us powerfully, for example the sun shines his light on us providing us with energy, vitality and life force. He (we will explain why the sun is a he later) brings the qualities of joy, happiness, confidence, self-empowerment, motivation and positivity. The sun inspires us to live our dreams, follow our goals and follow our individual calling, whatever that may be. The sun also sparks creativity, artistic and imaginative self-expression, and self-alignment to our purpose, destiny or true path. In Taoist philosophy and belief systems he is our will, our willpower and zest for life.

The moon, on the other hand, is our wisdom and emotional maturity. She (again, we explore this in-depth later) is our connection to our subconscious, all the shadow and hidden elements of self, and our subtle impressions, wishes and desires. The moon relates to our emotions, feelings, dreams, intuition, hidden fears and insecurities, wishes and inner desires. She is receptive in nature, unlike the sun who is assertive and active, and further speaks to us in silent yet powerful ways. We are strongly influenced by the moon for it is the moon's tides and energy currents that affect our feminine nature, and we all have a feminine nature. But this is especially true in women. The females of our species synchronize their own bodies' blood flow to that of the moon's- period blood is seen as a powerful life force energy to some cultures and traditions and the cycle itself is also known to many as a **moon cycle**. This one truth in itself shows just how connected we are to the planets in our orbit!

In dreams our subconscious, which is strongly influenced by the moon as mentioned, sends us messages, symbols and direct wisdom and insights. It is in dreams where we can be shown scenes, scenarios, visuals, and imagery into a number of life's problems. Through the powerful connection to the lunar energies of the moon the subconscious provides a type of mirror, allowing us to access those hidden and unseen parts of ourselves which can inevitably be learnt about and understood for healing and integration. Not only do dreams show us insight, wisdom, and messages into waking life, they also can directly show us aspects of our own selves in the form of shadows, emotions, traumas, and wounds holding us back. In this sense, the ability of the moon's subtle powers to influence in dream worlds combined with the sun's powers to profoundly affect us in waking life show just how powerful planets and astrological currents are at shaping, influencing, and affecting all living things on earth… Crystals are no different.

In addition to the sun and moon, below we explore some of the other main planets and how their subtle energies affect both us and crystals. We explore individual crystals in depth in later chapters, however, for now, let's have a look at the qualities associated with the planets in a more general and holistic way.

Mercury

Mercury is the messenger. He, being masculine in nature, is the planet of communication and has strong associations of the mind, intellect, and intelligence. Mercury in essence synthesizes information into connections, both neural and externally, as earth is an interconnected and living conscious entity. The energetic qualities associated with this planet are intuition, intellect, reasoning, thought, and cerebral explorations of mind. Anyone strongly influenced by Mercury therefore will most likely have great success in writing, speech, public speaking, and any career or hobby which relates to self-expression and communication. Any crystal which embodies the qualities of Mercury (has been strongly influenced by Mercury's astral energies during formation and development) can be used to enhance these elements, and can also aid in all aspects of learning mental processes. The key to remember, with all planets, is that their astral energies influence life on earth in some way. It is this astral energy which creates some of the healing and metaphysical properties in some crystals. We explore this throughout the rest of this book.

Crystals with a Mercurian influence: Blue Lace Agate, Sodalite, Sapphire, Amazonite, Amber, Lapis Lazuli, Aquamarine

Venus

Venus is the planet of love. She is feminine in nature and energy and relates to love, beauty, art, sensuality, love, romance and female sexuality. Venus' energy influences in many profound ways, from the types of relationships we have to our social and platonic interactions. She is responsible for our inner desires and feelings of love, romance, and intimacy. Desire and attraction are main themes with anyone strongly influenced by Venus, as is a strive towards peace, harmony, connection and beauty. Unlike Mars, her opposite, love and sex here are more erotic with wants and needs attuned to a more heart-centered and affectionate lust. Crystals which embody Venus' energy can therefore be used to greatly expand and develop all of the areas mentioned, in addition to bringing a sense of unconditional love and universal compassion.

Crystals with a Venian influence: Emerald, Jade, Tree Moss Agate, Ruby, Rhodonite, Rose Quartz, Citrine, Moonstone, Pearl

Mars

Mars is essentially Venus' counterpart. He too is a planet with strong energetic links to love, sex, and passion, yet he is symbolized by a more primal and aggressive lust. Will, action, assertion, and passion define him and- when expressed positively- the attributes of Mars can be very empowering. He is essentially ego and will in an ambitious and action-oriented way and therefore can result in some incredible self-learnings when connected to. Vitality, strength, and going after one's dreams can all be influenced by Mars. If balanced with the loving energy of Venus, this can also lead to some incredible advancements and developments in sexuality and sexual expression. Due to his association with being the planet of war and destruction he also has some very dark and destructive shadow elements, however. Any of the negative attributes associated with Mars therefore such as lust, anger, aggression, impulsiveness, impatience, insensitivity, and violence can all be healed and overcome with crystals which embody a more feminine and gentle energy, such as having association with Venus or water signs such as Pisces.

Crystals with a Martian influence: **Obsidian, Bloodstone**

Jupiter

Jupiter is our good luck planet. He brings optimism, good fortune, expansion, prosperity, and luck to anything he touches. He also relates to knowledge, philosophy, travel, adventure, wisdom, and higher consciousness. Jupiter is the planet which can help us understand the connection between spirituality, the energetic universe we live in, and the physical world. His energetic and metaphysical characteristics which profoundly affect us can be seen to match his physical manifestation. This is because Jupiter is one of the larger planets, therefore it is no surprise that he represents expansion, good fortune, and luck. He also brings abundance and material manifestation and, as you will see later, the crystals which embody the qualities of Jupiter can lead to great healing, shifts in vibration, and self-development.

Crystals with Jupiterian energy: Topaz, Aventurine, Carnelian, Peacock Ore, Tiger's Eye, Turquoise, Amber, Citrine, Amethyst

Saturn

Saturn is the way shower. In ancient mythology, he is known as 'Father Time' due to his energetic associations of limitation, structure, and conservation. Saturn brings a karmic quality and element to his influence, as he has strong links to the collective shadow and a need to structure, discipline, and set boundaries. This naturally creates a karmic element as we humans naturally desire freedom, soul expression, and liberation from ties and responsibilities which may hold us down. Yet Saturn does exactly this. He brings wisdom, maturity, and great responsibility, and sometimes to vast extents of duties and restrictions. In its positive expression, however, the energies of Saturn and crystals associated can bring great maturity, inner-healing, wisdom, and growth. Stability and teaching important lessons in duty, responsibility, and karma are paramount.

Crystals with Saturnian energy: Black Tourmaline, Red Jasper, Hematite

Uranus

Uranus is the awakener. He represents the dualistic nature of both human nature and reality and can therefore lead to transformation, genius, invention, and liberation. The energy associated is often one of change, originality and vibration, initially manifesting as some sort of chaos and break down to lead to invention and transformation. In its negative aspect,

Uranus is rebellious; there is a desire to transcend limits and move beyond boundaries. This can of course be positive. For example, working with crystals which lead to innovation, invention, shifting old paradigms, and introducing new ways of thinking and independence can have great effects. Essentially, Uranus embodies a higher vibration energy. Being conscious of his energy when working crystals therefore can lead to great transformation and shifts in vibration.

Crystals with Uranian energy: Smoky Quartz, Garnet, Fluorite, Labradorite, Azurite

Neptune

Neptune is the visionary planet of astrology. Energetic associations include inspiration, ecstasy, illusion, mysticism, fantasy, and high levels of creative or artistic expression. There is an urge to transcend with Neptune, flying past the ordinary to create something extraordinary and tune in to some higher power, idea, or new artistic creation. Poets, artists, musicians, deep thinkers, philosophers, creatives, and dreamers are associated with Neptunian energy; as are visionaries, spiritual leaders, or teachers. Neptune also embodies the vibration of unconditional love and can lead to ecstasy and enlightenment when connected to. In its negative association, however, Neptune can lead to fantasy, escapism, delusion, and addictions such as drugs, substance, alcohol, or sex.

Crystals with Neptunian energy: Tree Moss Agate, Blue Lace Agate, Aquamarine, Carnelian, Amazonite, Amethyst, Ruby, Azurite, Pyrite, Lapis Lazuli, Turquoise, Sugilite, Selenite, Celestite

Pluto

Pluto's energies relate to life, death, and rebirth; the cyclic nature of existence. He represents regeneration, rebirth, and destruction leading to new and improved energy or qualities. Pluto seeks to destroy in a way which brings healing, cleansing, and new life. Interestingly, Pluto has a strong association with Scorpio, the star sign, and Scorpio itself is the sign strongly associated with death and rebirth. This planet is also associated with darkness and unresolved or repressed issues such as resentments, jealousies, envies, and destructive feelings and thoughts. Because of this, Pluto can have a very positive and powerful effect when utilized constructively, specifically through its characteristics of regeneration, rebirth, and purification. Crystals with a strong plutonian energy often embody power and a sense of transformation, or access to higher consciousness.

Crystals with Plutonian energy: Bloodstone, Lapis Lazuli, Jade, Garnet, Labradorite, Amethyst, Peacock Ore

Chiron

It would be wise to mention Chiron, the Wounded healer. Chiron is more an asteroid than a planet, however, as with all entities and conscious bodies of energy in space, we are still influenced by him here on earth. Chiron represents the wound of the soul. He is the cosmic messenger who can show us what and where we need to heal and what we may still unconsciously be holding on to. Like with other planets Chiron has strong links to the shadow, those wounded and hidden parts of ourselves within. People strongly affected by Chiron make excellent nurses, doctors, healers, therapists, counselors, and carers, as they can use their own inner wounds and life's traumas to help others. Chiron is a beautiful example of the strength of the human spirit as Chriron himself used his own experience and wounds to be of service and healing to others.

Crystals with energy relating to Chiron: Malachite, Amethyst, Sapphire, Selenite, Rhodonite

It is important to note that we are all influenced by the planets, however to varying degrees. Just like people are more affected by the sun's rays than others and women and some are more affected by the moon's subtle energy, the same is true for all of the planets. It is important when working with crystals therefore, to be aware of how astrological transits and bodies may be influencing us. It is often the behind the scenes, subtle vibrations which have a profound effect on all aspects of our lives. Of course, crystals work on an energetic, subtle, and metaphysical level, implying that looking to the stars and planets may aid in our journey of transformation and accessing new states of consciousness and vibration mastery.

Crystal Spirit & Science

Spirit science is a term you may find yourself adopting the more familiar you become with crystals and their use. Everything has a spirit just as everything can be measured by science. Simultaneously, science defines us just as everything can be seen to hold a spiritual-energetic essence. Regardless of whether you are more scientifically minded or possessing a spiritual perspective, spirit and science are both fundamental parts to the understanding and integration of crystals. Why, you may be asking? Because; even when we begin to experience the first-hand effects of crystals and their healing properties, going so far into spirituality and esotericism is counterproductive to the self. We have both a right brain and left brain and ultimately, they wish to be unified. Working with crystals and harnessing their energy therefore balances them. Greater awareness, intuition, and perception to subtle energy is increased, yet so is our sense of groundedness and being connected to the earth. This is why all those schools of thoughts or predominantly left-brain scientific minds have got it wrong. Crystals aren't some 'woo' or hippy, away with the fairies nonsense; they are very real and deeply powerful natural entities which can help us in so many ways. In Chapter 2, we explore these ways.

Chapter 2: How Crystals Work

By now, you can probably begin to realize exactly how important it is to balance your chakras. While researchers are still studying links between the spiritual, emotional, mental, and physical realms, the chakra system is backed by thousands of years of practice. Innumerable people across decades and all parts of the world have found that taking proper care to maintain their chakras is an effective way to boost mental and physical health and to combat serious issues.

In fact, many of the potential issues listed above that can result from imbalanced chakras seem quite frightening - you probably didn't know that diseases found in major organs could be affected by something like your energy field. Yet, it makes sense - after all, each of us is made up of energy, and the way in which our energy reacts with that of our surroundings naturally has an effect on us.

Of course, sometimes this effect can be positive, but in many cases, the toxins and negative energy sources we're exposed to have a detrimental effect on us.

That's why crystals are so important. Despite efforts to eat clean, reduce your carbon footprint, or exercise regularly, your chakras still need an extra boost to be perfectly regulated. Healing crystals hold the key to unlocking unlimited wellness potential within your mind and body.

It seems crazy, probably, to anyone who isn't familiar with the concept. How could a rock possibly have any sort of healing processes? We'll explain.

As we mentioned above, the most important aspect of balancing your chakras is ensuring the fact that their vibratory frequencies are resonating at their ideal levels. An irregularity can occur from a disturbance, which causes the vibratory pattern to be thrown off.

Consequently, we feel out of sorts, either in mental or physical capacity, or both. Healing crystals, then, have the capacity to regulate these patterns and restore harmony within our chakras.

To explain it simply, crystals, like all other aspects of our world, have their own distinct vibratory patterns. Yet, healing crystals emit some of the purest resonances, thanks to their innate, balanced structure. The vibrations they offer our chakras act as tuning forks, bringing our energy field back to the level at which it vibrates most efficiently, thereby restoring health and harmony. Yet, you must allow yourself to be mentally, physically, and spiritually receptive to these restorations, which can be an issue for some nonbelievers.

To anyone who discredits the value of healing crystals, it's important to understand that there is, in fact, a scientific facet to this practice. Think of it this way: it's a known fact that despite the classifications of gasses, liquids, and solids, nothing is ever truly wholly "solid;" rather, anything that's solid is made up of a series of moving atoms, in addition to molecules and minerals. Thus, the atoms that are moving among us have an energy about them.

People, therefore, are complex beings, made up of energy fields that embody nature's balance and organizational properties. Just as our chakra patterns are unique, so, too, is each crystal. The pattern at which each stone resonates corresponds best with specific chakras. To heal ourselves holistically, we can choose certain crystals to best harmonize the chakras among us that may have experienced an imbalance. Each crystal is an active participant in nature with a valuable purpose.

Chapter 3: Crystal Therapists

A crystal energy healing therapist will treat the affected chakras by placing, or sometimes rubbing, specific types of crystals oven the chakras in question. Interestingly enough, there's no such thing as "one crystal-fits-all." Therapists will have a variety of crystals, and will decide which crystals need to be used, based on the answers you supply to their questions.

Crystal healing experiences also vary from one individual to the next, although it's not uncommon for people to say it feels as though a huge load has been lifted off their shoulders. Many also report a distinctive tingling sensation, which varies depending on the severity of the blockage or blockages regarding the various chakras. While no two people have the same experience and while some see better results than others, all agree that in order to really benefit from crystal healing, one has to maintain an open mind.

The physics principle behind the magic

Advocates for Crystal Healing have been around for centuries. Most people have and do assume that it is quackery. But a research project found the scientific mechanism that allows our body's energy field to receive transmissions from radiating crystals. Crystal Healing is not quackery.

The Third Eye:

The ancient Third Eye of our ancestors had been designed to receive external vibrations of various frequencies, including light. It has evolved down through the ages to become our pineal gland. It now secretes the melatonin hormone that controls our daily lives.

The research shows how it enables our human body to receive external vibrations such as the soothing frequencies of certain crystals.

Of the several types of crystals studied it was found that the amethyst crystal had the best measurable energy field with the most available data, so most of the evaluations were on the amethyst crystal.

A key to understanding the science can perhaps best be recognized from Einstein's famous equation $E=MC^2$ which shows that our bodies are basically two kinds of matrices: one of matter (M) which is our flesh and bone, and one of energy (E) which has a measurable electromagnetic field. (C is the speed of light.) Advocates of Crystal Healing call this electromagnetic field our aura.

The basic research objective was then to find a mechanism that could enable our bodies to receive an energy transmission from a radiating crystal. This is where chakras and auras come into play.

Chakras:

Chakra is an old Sanskrit term meaning 'wheel' or 'circle' and is used to reference

7 specific energy centers along the body's meridian. Note that the Brow Chakra is also known as the Third Eye and this is the one of most importance in the research.

Our western philosophy does not generally consider Chakras as anything more than unfounded myths from the ancient world.

Most Americans dismiss the idea of chakras as notions resurrected by the "new-age movement". But we know that the idea of chakras goes back many thousands of years.

The earliest mention of Chakras comes from the Vedas that form the Hindu scriptures. Evidence indicates that the Vedas were brought to pre-historical India when the early founders migrated from a lost civilization. Plato said that civilization was Atlantis.

The Chakras are said to be "force centers" in the physical body that are occupied by whorls of energy. Their energy may also radiate from these points in the physical body.

Chakras are basically accepted as symbolic, however many people believe them to be physical. To understand how chakras might be physical, it's important to remember that energy is physical, and chakras are believed to be discs of energy. Remember that the electricity in our nervous systems and brainwaves is energy.

It is believed that the Brow Chakra which is known as the Third Eye is the most important from a Crystal Healing standpoint. In analyzing this Third Eye we see that our ancient ancestors did indeed have a Third Eye that could sense vibrations from their environment. Some primitive creatures still living today, such as the Mantis and Iguana have Third Eyes.

The advocates claim that Crystal Healing is a deep and gentle healing technique that is very effective. The technique is to focus the energy from specific crystals onto the patient's Chakras and Aura Field. The energy is focused at the points where the Chakras and Aura that may need "balancing" are most sensitive.

The advocates claim that our Chakras and Auras control the energy flow into every area of our lives.

Each chakra has a specific significance in that each, with one exception, relates to a gland in the endocrine system.

Auras:

The aura is the electromagnetic field that surrounds the human body and every organism and object in the Universe. This is a true and undisputed scientific fact.

But some devotees of Crystal Healing also believe that auras can show if someone is highly spiritual or may be interacting with another entity. The devotees also believe that auras show the well being of the person giving off the aura. They believe that the aura colors of a person indicate specific aspects of the person. Remember that each color is a specific spectrum of frequencies, or vibrations.

Silver indicates intelligence, Ruby Red indicates vitality, Violet indicates gentleness, Rose Pink indicates love, Sapphire Blue indicates healing and spirituality, Gray indicates illness or fear, Brown indicates cruelty or stubbornness.

How crystal energy works and later discovery

The evidence shows that our Third Eye (our pineal gland) can sense the energy field of some perfect or near perfect crystals.

To understand how this works we need to recognize that our bodies are energy matrixes; that amethyst Crystals are energy matrixes and that the two energy fields can interact via our Third Eye.

Let's visualize the interaction of energy vibrations from a crystal with the energy vibrations in our human electromagnetic field. The interaction of the uniform crystal vibrations tends to sooth the body's aura into a more peaceful order. That is the essence of crystal healing.

Mind-Body Connection

Research found the scientific mechanism that allows our body's energy field to receive transmissions from radiating crystals.

The ancient Third Eye of our ancestors has evolved such that it can help receive external vibrations such as the soothing frequencies of certain crystals.

Healing properties of crystals

You may find it hard to believe, but crystals and minerals DO actually have healing properties. Although the science is not well understood, there is plenty of people, cultures, and history that advocate the use of particular crystals and gems for particular uses. Allow me to explain the basics.

Have you ever slept with a crystal under your pillow? Try it using amethyst or malachite and you will notice an obvious affect on your dreams. Open up to the idea that crystals can help heal your mental, physical, emotional, and/or spiritual state. Once you do, you will have a new hope and a new method for practical self-improvement through crystal healing.

Most Americans these days only believe in proven science. Well, everything IS science, but only some of it has been proven. Take our thoughts for an example. We all have thoughts, but we still can't read them or prove them with scientific instruments. Here we get the "gray area" of Metaphysics. So, to believe in Crystals that Heal, you must understand that Metaphysics is science not yet proven. We still don't have sensitive enough equipment to measure the higher activities of crystals and minerals. Plus, we're not looking for it.

How do crystals heal, then? By subtly altering our Vibrational patterns. Have you ever seen Dr. Emoto's water experiments? Science has proven that all matter is actually energy and all energy vibrates. Science has also proven that thoughts, prayers, and other surprising things can alter those energy vibrations. Crystals hold a vibrational pattern that affects the frequencies and vibrations of water as well as those of people (and their bio-electro-magnetic field.)

Different crystals and minerals hold different Vibrational patterns, so by utilizing different gemstones, you can affect different parts of your physical, emotional, mental, and/or spiritual anatomy. The longer you are exposed to a particular type of crystal, the more it can have an impact on you, as your vibrational patterns naturally align with the crystal's vibrational patterns.

Understanding that the vibrations of minerals and gemstones are about as fine as those of thoughts and emotions, is easy to see why believing in the Healing Power of Crystals would increase their potency. And so does wearing or holding a crystal right up against the skin or ingesting a Gemstone Elixir (where you are drinking water that has had a crystal soaking in it - thereby altering the waters molecular structure just as thoughts alter water molecules in the Dr. Emoto Research.) The length of time that a person is in contact with a crystal is also a factor in how much impact the crystal will have.

Shape, Color, and Grids

Crystals you should know

There's been a in American adults turning to what's known as complementary and alternative medicine. This includes everything from acupuncture and yoga to tai chi and even healing crystals.

In fact, you've probably heard people talking about, and showing off, these beautiful stones. But you may not know what they could offer you.

There are a number of different types of crystals, each filled with their own healing abilities for the mind, body, and soul. They're thought to promote the flow of good energy and help rid the body and mind of negative energy for physical and emotional benefits.

Historically speaking, crystals are touted as ancient forms of medicine, with philosophies borrowed from Hinduism and Buddhism. However, it's important to know that there's no scientific evidence to support the use of crystals. Despite this, people are still drawn to their colors and beauty.

The key to indulging in this self-care experience is mindfulness, reflection, and acceptance. For instance, found that a person's mind may have much more healing power than it's given credit.

Even though there isn't a great deal of scientific support of crystals, a number of people swear by their powers. So, if you're curious to give them a go, make sure to keep an open mind and check out what each stone can do for you.

To help you get started, we compiled a comprehensive roundup of some of the most popular crystals.

Chapter 4: How To Prepare For Natural And Manmade Disasters

One of the main purposes of keeping a healing crystal is protection. There is no limitation to what a crystal can protect. Different crystals offer defenses against a variety of problems and disasters. For example, certain crystals can be used to mentally prepare for natural and manmade disasters. Individuals can use crystals to eliminate negative energies both within the individual and in the environment. The following crystals are known for such protection powers:

Amber

Smoky Quartz

Black Tourmaline

Green Tourmaline

Aqua

Sapphire

Rutilated Quartz

Black Onyx

Hematite

Garnet

Amethyst

Protective Circle

The only way to protect yourself and your home from both natural and manmade disasters with crystals is by creating a protective circle around your house. The protective circle keeps your house safe from all that you fear. Whether it is fear of burglary or a storm, you will be able to free yourself from all of it simply by using your crystals. The best aspect of this practice is the permanent nature of the circle.

Making a protective circle does not require mastery in the crystal healing process. The process is rather simple to understand and reciprocate. The ritual is also executed indoors. All that one needs to establish a protective circle is a protection crystal and a sage bundle. Sage is used for cleansing purposes, cleansing the entire space of any unnecessary or harmful energies. The crystal adds to the protection established by the sage.

The first step is centering: You need to center and ground yourself before beginning the ritual. Second, light the sage bundle and blow on the bundle until it smokes. Once the bundle begins to smoke, hold the sage bundle in your hands and walk around the entire space that needs protection, in a counter-clockwise direction. Make sure the smoke reaches each corner of each room and the space above and below the windows and doors.

The next step involves using your protection crystal. Try using a large stone for this. Program the crystal for protection by keeping it in your left hand and using your right hand to cover the top of the crystal and announce your purpose. For example, you can announce that you are dedicating the stone to the protection of your house. Then, simply walk around the space in the same path while holding the crystal.

Protective shields

A protective shield can also be created around the house by playing with the positions of protective crystals. You can place crystals at each corner of the home, creating an external shield for your entire house.

Additionally, crystals have the ability to protect individuals from both personal and environmental negative energies. The electromagnetic fields from technology around your house such as the computer and television can be neutralized by placing a crystal such as Fluorite near them. Geographic stress can be absorbed by crystals like Smoky Quartz. Human-based negative energies can be neutralized by using Amber or a Bloodstone.

These crystals can be an amazing stress reliever for the workplace as well. You can simply place a smoky Quartz on your office desk to defend yourself against stress projected by other people.

Chapter 5: How Crystal Healing Works

Crystals are living stones that have been present on Earth since the very beginning of time. Crystals have been used in healing since the start of civilization. Crystals are used to heal physical, mental, emotional, and spiritual problems.

According to metaphysics, crystals can transform us. The tough part of crystal healing is figuring out which crystals to use for healing. For most cases, the color of the crystal is an indicator as to what type of healing it can be used for. For example, white stones are used for healing spiritual problems.

There are different types of stones and crystals that are used for healing and each of them works in a different way. Some of the larger stones can also be used for cleansing of the crystals. Wands are used extensively in meditation and organ specific healing. All stones are found naturally on Earth and hence are charged with energy from Earth.

Crystals have extra electrons that are stored within their lattices. It is these electrons that allow crystals to change one form of energy into another. When a crystal is heated or subjected to pressure, it alters its form and transforms itself into another stone. This energy can be harnessed to heal a person.

Energy is the basic essence of a human. Each crystal has its own type of energy. When crystals are used to heal, the energy from the crystal blends with the energy from the body thereby amplifying the energy within the body. It aids in rebalancing the energy within the body. Crystals can change the way we think.

Since the energy from the crystal is used to heal a person's body, it is better if the crystal is adjusted to the person who needs the healing.

The reason why crystals have a positive and soothing effect on our bodies is because of the many metaphysical properties that they possess.

Crystals help in reenergizing our bodies at the physical, mental, spiritual, and emotional levels. They help in purifying our minds and bodies. They align these four energy levels and maintain a balance.

They help in maintaining a balance between the Yin and Yang. Yin and Yang are considered to be opposing forces with the Yin being the feminine and the Yang being the masculine. Crystals stabilize these two and maintain equilibrium in our aura.

Crystals are used to improve concentration and also to clear the third eye during meditation. They help in increasing intuition. They are also used to improve communication and instill strength and courage in a person.

Chapter 6: Everyday Uses For Healing Crystals

Precious stones and gemstones are to be utilized in mix with current medication; never use these instead of medicinal treatment. If you are debilitated or harmed, at that point you should see a specialist right away. These items are used to help improve your energy and this can help in the mending procedure.

Science will in general markdown anything that it can't clarify. Numerous individuals have been recuperated on confidence alone. If this is conceivable, at that point, positive energy may help in mending also. Some may even say that similar conviction that recuperated an individual was a type of this energy moved to start with one individual then onto the next.

These may not work for every single individual. There may be restrictions just as conceivable obstruction, for example, when the stone is encompassed by metal. This is probably the primary motivation why these have been limited by science; they don't have similar outcomes every single time or for every single individual who attempts to utilize this sort of treatment.

The general standard is that precious stones and gemstones have an energy all their own. When you wear these, at that point that power might be moved to you. Your bodies energy may then be adjusted regardless of whether somewhat. This can invigorate you and speed the mending procedure. This is much a similar rule as nourishment giving the body energy aside from this is from an outside source.

Numerous kinds of gems and gemstones can be utilized for this sort of treatment. Some are of a lot higher quality, and it is regularly accepted that the better the nature of gemstone then the better the energy from that stone. There are numerous sites accessible which can enable you to figure out what properties various stones may have and how to pick the best stones.

No one but you can see whether mending precious stones are directly for you. There are reports of these mending wounds, sickness, and even in getting out from under negative behavior patterns like smoking. Check whether this kind of treatment is directly for you today and you may be more advantageous tomorrow.

Using Healing Crystals

Individuals have utilized crystals for recuperating for a large number of years. Recuperating diamonds have not exclusively been used for medicinal reasons all through the ages, yet for enchantment, assurance, customs, and cash. Today, many keep on utilizing recuperating crystals to upgrade their prosperity.

Kinds of mending crystals

Each mending precious stone has a different arrangement of one of a kind properties. For instance, clear quartz is said to improve your safe framework. The features of moonstone incorporate enhancing the intensity of your instinct. Tiger's eye can help quiet your nerves and lift your fearlessness. When you are inclined to bad dreams, amethyst is known to offer assistance. Remember that any metals that touch crystals, including silver, can decrease the crystals' quality, if not making them inadequate.

Utilizing mending crystals

All together for mending crystals to be best, the glasses ought to be cleaned, charged, and modified. You can cleanse your crystals in a few different ways, for example, leaving them in the sun, placing them in salt water or covering them in the ground. Cleaning your crystals will expel any undesirable or pointless vitality that the glasses developed through taking care of before you got them.

To charge your crystals and give them a lift, leave them outside under the light of a full moon throughout the night. When you make the most of your glasses and don't have a specific reason as the main priority for them, you don't have to program your stones. When you need to utilize your crystals for a particular purpose, you may sit, hold your glasses, and imagine what you might want from them. This is the easiest method to program crystals.

You may believe that holding a precious stone or wearing a gem is the main ways that crystals can be utilized. This isn't the situation. Diamonds can be held under cushions or put in your tub when you are cleaning up. Glasses kept at workspaces can add positive vitality to your day just as balance the electrical impacts of electrical necessities, for example, PCs and artificial lighting. You can utilize diamond water, which you can make by leaving a precious stone in spring water for ten hours, by pouring it in your bath, spritzing it on your body or drinking it.

Chakras Healing Crystals

A chakra is a vortex or turning arrangement of vitality, which identifies with a specific recurrence or capacity.

HOW Can IT WORK?

The vitality comes into this reality and leaves employing the chakras. Each chakra speaks to a bit of the range, and together all the chakras make one entire being as they turn.

The vitality from our soul or unadulterated cognizance ventures itself upon this reality. As it comes in it structures two segments - the inward reality, the three upper chakras and the external, (the physical), the three lower chakras, with the heart chakra being the middle, transformational or parity point.

The chakras turn and attract vitality or out as indicated by our needs. They move the spirit and rearrange it as per the change procedure for this life.

A gem is a strong vitality structure that transmits a specific recurrence. Chakra recuperating crystals can empower us to entrain to energies inside them, and these energies can assist us with healing, balance, and change our bodies, psyches, and emotions. We should know

We started to free the capacity to recollect our identity because of all the "stuff" or static vitality we curb. This fills and obstructs the lower chakras. It happens because we prop up additional into our brains, never truly being in our lives, at this time. The lower chakras slowly fill with stuff, since we were not here in our lives to be with and change it on the spot. This squares us in knowing our untouched nature and reality of our identity. Anyway, it is all piece of the jigsaw astounds of our helping procedure. Truth be told nothing is excellent or bad......it is merely.

How to Use Crystals

Utilizing precious stones can completely change you. There 'is regardless, just vitality,' he told our reality what such enormous numbers of vitality laborers knew. Everything is made of vitality that vibrates at various frequencies and paces. Our body, our psyche, even our feelings are on the inclusive rates that are continually evolving. We can influence these energies or frequencies from numerous points of view, and we can make them more grounded, flimsier parity them, or irregularity them — each idea, development, what we eat, our identity changes minute by minute. Recuperating with precious stones can empower us to re-arrange and re-balance the energies of our body, brain, condition, and feelings.

When we are realizing 'how to utilize gems,' we have to consider the vitality they hold and what we are needing to accomplish through utilizing them. Most 'precious stones' hold at least one frequencies, we can think about how everyone can influence every one of our many energies, or we can figure out how to utilize gems intuitively. This is significantly more dominant than having many books we need to paw through. Precious stones that hold more than one mineral or gem type give us more for our cash and amplify the intensity of the gem. Like when we contain gold, silver, copper, pyrite iron in blanketed quartz. This implies they hold many adjusting transformational frequencies and are ideal for utilizing as gem recuperating stones.

First, you need to 'become more acquainted with' your precious stones. Gems will tell you the best way to recuperate with precious jewels when you let them direct you. Convey them with you and sit in some cases quietly in a peaceful spot and hold back to feel their vitality, the shivering, the glow or cool or any messages from them. Give them a chance to turn into your companion, be guided concerning where your hand appears to need to put them. Go with your first inclination about to what extent they should be there. "Premonitions' are typically right. Your precious stone mending stones can assist you with balancing your energies as you get more 'tuned in to them and the vitality they convey.

They can turn into your 'pet,' and you can find that they are an incredible help to you. They should be washed down consistently except if they hold adjusting minerals like gold inside them.

To rinse a precious stone, applaud over it and after that grin into it, you could likewise run it under virus water and spot it in the sun.

'Precious stones' can be an astounding tool in our life. Keep in mind precious stones are incredible blessings.

Instructions to Use Crystal Healing Wands

Precious stone wands are not ordinarily framed commonly. Single point eliminators will some of the time be adjusted on the base, yet as a rule, they are cut from bigger gem squares. Changing the bottom enables it to be utilized as a back rub tool straightforwardly on the skin. You can use gem wands to ease pressure anyplace in the body. They function admirably on the head, feet, and hands.

Another utilization for a precious stone recuperating wands is checking the atmosphere to distinguish blockages The Crystal Wand can be utilized to expel the obstruction in various ways.

As Quartz Crystal is both Piezoelectric and Pyroelectric, you can change the extremity of the gem when it is exposed to either weight or warmth. The tip will abandon being typically positive and getting too cynical, thus transmitting vitality from the tip. I have discovered this is valuable when taking a shot at a specific area, you can gather the energy in a tight shaft, thus amplify the recuperating area.

I have utilized mending wands in various ways and an assortment of gem types. Again be guided by your instinct and not by what others state is correct or wrong.

To filter the quality pursue the strategy beneath (again you can change the technique when you feel the need).

1. Take the wand in your dominant hand, holding the point towards the customer.

2. Pick a beginning stage and start moving the precious stone wand gradually around the body, making a note of any areas that vibe extraordinary.

3. Now and again, you may feel that the mending wand it challenging to move, at times it will vibrate marginally. These emotions, for the most part, demonstrate blockages.

4. After you have wrapped up the quality, return, and work on the blocked areas,

utilizing either the precious stone wand or any recuperating gems that you feel essential.

Again let your instinct guide you; there is no set in a stone manner to do this.

Use Crystals For Healing

Alternative ways to deal with drug flourish for the individuals who are searching for another approach to treat their sickness or condition. Precious stones have been utilized for a long time to direct vitality to the patient who is searching for amending or advantage from the rock. Science has not demonstrated or decided how stones direct vitality, however plainly energy goes through gems in an arranged and understandable way. When you are utilizing precious stones for your own recuperating, it is significant that you get master data on the assortment of ways that they can be used.

Utilizing gems during reflection is an exceptionally well-known approach to use the stones. Numerous individuals hold the stones during consideration to enable the vitality to move through them and help them recuperate any physical issues that they may have. Others will put the precious rocks and stones directly on the body in the territory where they are experiencing difficulty.

Various stones are utilized in gem treatment. The multiple stones are being used for an assortment of purposes. When you are looking into the utilization of gems, pay particular consideration regarding the rocks that are used in your treatment. There are numerous assets of this data on the web, and you can peruse how the stones can be utilized for your very own treatment.

Significantly, you counsel with your primary care physician when you are confronting an ailment or ailment. The utilization of precious stones is anything but a substitute for reasonable restorative consideration. You ought to consistently examine your arrangements for alternative prescription with your primary care physician to make sure that you are not causing an issue with your conventional treatment.

Ensure that you do your exploration on the utilization of gems for mending and wellbeing. You need to make sure that you are getting the ideal data on how and when you should utilize these precious stones in your treatment plan. There can be a medical advantage, yet you ought not to ignore the treatment of conventional prescription when you are confronting a genuine medical problem. Science has not demonstrated or refuted the utilization of precious stones for your wellbeing, and you may make issues your wellbeing if you choose to set aside common medications that could profit you for gem treatment.

Alternative prescription works best when it is utilized related to other treatment choices. Examine your treatment alternatives with your primary care physician and ensure that you are using the best open doors that you have accessible to you to treat and fix your ailment.

The most effective method to Cleanse Crystals

The gemstone vitality medication development reemerged decades back with enthusiasm for gems for recuperating and precious stone groups for inspiring the vibrations of rooms. If recuperating stones are appropriately thought about, their capacities are broad. At the point when connected restoratively, gems help discharge unwanted energies from the patient's body and emanation. In time, these unwanted energies gather on the precious stones' surface just as in the vitality field that encompasses them. Much like the messiness on a work area can hinder your capacity to work, the undesirable energies on a gem impede its mending powers, and the stones must be purified.

If you use precious stone groups in your home or office to help keep the room's climate clear and elevated, purge the gems each time you dust, or about once consistently or two. This will enable them to work taking care of business. Mending precious stones ought to be purified after each treatment session wherein you use them. When you don't wash down your precious stones as proposed, three outcomes may happen. To start with, negative energies that the mending gems get could be transmitted to the following individual who receives the treatment. Second, you, as the specialist, may unwittingly get these energies. At long last, the gem may keep on retaining the unwanted powers, which will further cloud the precious stone, making it less viable as a recuperating apparatus.

Fortunately, precious stones react particularly well to purifying. Begin by cleaning your recuperating precious rocks with water. This will expel the residue and soil that amasses on the precious stones' surface. Utilize running water from your sink just if your faucet water is non-chlorinated. You will likewise require an old toothbrush and some gentle cleanser or cleanser. Hold your precious stones under the running water, put some detergent on the toothbrush, and brush the gem surfaces.

While the cleanser evacuates the physical earth and residue from the gems, the movement of the running water expels unwanted energies your recuperating precious stones may have gotten during therapeutic use, or while keeping the vitality in a room inspired and clear. If your faucet water is dealt with, empty some cleaned water into an enormous estimating cup or pitcher. Purge the precious stones with the lathery toothbrush as in the past, but instead than utilizing your spigot, wash them by pouring the cleansed water over them.

When the precious stones are physically washed down, you can likewise clear their vitality field utilizing a pearl formula vitality removing purging spray. This will take out unwanted energies that the vitality field may have gotten.

While utilizing cleanser and running water over your gems is viable for evacuating unwanted energies, this technique isn't successful in clearing electromagnetic radiation (EMR) that the precious stones may have grabbed from a patient's body and atmosphere during a treatment session. Precious stones can likewise ingest EMR from situations with high electromagnetic fields. A pearl formula EMR protection spray was intended to deal with this circumstance. Spray your precious stones with this formula to free them of electromagnetic radiation.

Next, spray your precious stones with a pearl formula jewel mending restoring spray. This will clear collected vitality from the precious stones' diagrams to achieve forward data their actual reason. You, as the specialist, can naturally choose the good ways from the precious stones to hold the spray, and furthermore at what point. The more cautiously you tweak the spray rinse, the more powerful it will be.

By utilizing both cleanser and water to clean your gems physically, and diamond formula sprays to clear them vigorously, your precious stones will probably express their most extreme mending potential.

The Types of Crystals Used in Crystal Chandeliers

Crystal ceiling fixtures are maybe the best embellishments you can ever adorn your homes with. Since they are hanged up high in the roof, they can be adequately valued by guests coming in your home. Furthermore, because they are crystal made, they sparkle like no other fancy piece in your home.

In picking crystal ceiling fixtures, you should be skilled with an eye for the crystal. Since this is the fundamental fascination in the light fixture, it must be ideal enough for your homes. Before buying these lighting installations, you have to think well about the sorts of crystals utilized in ceiling fixtures. Doing as such would mean picking the ideal crystal light fixture for home use.

The Swarovski Crystal

Swarovski is the best crystal on the planet. It began in Austria where the most lovely crystal pieces are conceived. It is said that the Swarovski crystal is as bright as the spring water. It has remarkable splendor and magnificence which a gem ought to have. The Swarovski crystal is additionally accessible in numerous hues. There are silver, gold, and other crystal hues with mirror-like quality. Today, Swarovski is utilized in multiple crystal light fixtures as a result of the undetectable covering around it that takes into consideration more straightforward cleaning.

Handcut Crystals

Handcut crystals ooze in quality. They experience several procedures before a bit of diamond is at long last made. Others utilize the legacy strategy where the crystal suffers specific slices through iron and sandstone wheel. Optical glasses, then again, include the utilization of sure modern gear which is amazingly refractive.

Inheritance Crystals

If you lean toward crystals produced using Venice, at that point the Legacy crystal is ideal for you. Their glasses are shaped and fire-cleaned as opposed to being cut. Typically, Venetian glasses offer an antique look in homes. Most planners today lean toward this sort of crystal for an increasingly real intrigue.

Vintage Crystals

Vintage crystals are the ones, for the most part, found in antique accumulations. Beside the glass itself, the light fixture is enhanced with dots and other vintage structures. Whimsical gems are additionally incorporated into the ceiling fixtures to make an increasingly offbeat feel. Oval shaped antique pieces, dainty beads, and even octagon shaped crystal pieces are incorporated into the Vintage kind of crystal light fixture.

Shake Crystal

When you lean toward a progressively old look in your homes, at that point, the stone sort of crystal light fixture would do well as an inside adornment. Each stone crystal takes billions of years to frame. That is the reason, each stone crystal piece you'll get is in reality exceptionally one of a kind. It can't be replicated or duplicated since just one of its own exists. With a climate you are in, the stone crystal is cool to contact. In spite of its being the rock in highlight, it makes a baffling coolness on it and the earth encompassing it.

Different Types of Crystals and How to Use Them

Precious stones are accessible in the market in such a large number of various sizes, shapes, and hues. Individuals frequently get befuddled, considering which precious stones they should utilize. Some of them even begin wearing gems without checking whether it will genuinely suit their zodiac sign. These precious stones ought to be chosen by zodiac signs so it will profit you and your wellbeing, because picking an off-base gem may influence your wellbeing as well as change your social and expert life.

It isn't fundamental that you need to wear these precious stones to pick up something from them, you can likewise experience specific gem recuperating treatment sessions and consequently, for that, you ought to know for which chakra a particular flower is utilized. There are in each of the seven chakras in our body which are otherwise called vitality discharging focuses. These chakras ought to be refined to dispose of all the negative energies and ailments. This procedure helps in adjusting the progression of vitality in the individual's body. The healer who is doing the recuperating system on somebody should initially experience the act of gem mending to make his body unadulterated and free from any negative vitality. This vitality would then be able to be moved from his body to someone else through the gems. Like this, the individual experiencing any disease brought about by the negative vitality will be relieved.

There are various sorts of gems which are utilized in the gem mending process. They are:

1. Amethyst: This gem is identified with eyes, hair, scalp, adjusting glucose, migraines, pituitary organ, and furthermore in lessening outrage.

2. Sea green/blue: Related to the safe system, lymph nodes, flexibility, innocence, creativity, joy, communication, self-knowledge, fear, anxiety, and certainty.

3. Carnelian: Related to kidneys, feelings, sexuality, reproductive system, issues, menstrual, joint inflammation, nerve bladder, decisiveness, and pancreas.

4. Coral: Related to blood, muscles, reproductive systems, metabolism, thyroid, heart, to make your feelings more grounded, and it ought to be carefully kept away from by the individual having hypertension.

5. Citrine: Related to nourishment issue, kidneys, liver, hypersensitivities, mental and enthusiastic, digestion tracts, tension, sorrow, fear, self-discipline, memory, causticity, critical thinking, and so on.

6. Jade: Related to Immune system, thymus, heart, sensory system, kidney, knowledge, mental fortitude, enthusiastic parity, riches, congruity, life span, empathy, equity, and cleaning of blood.

7. Precious stone: Related to trust, love, success, shortcoming, and quality, expanding own clarity, certainty, mentalities, and otherworldliness.

8. Lapis: Related to eagerness, bashfulness, discourse, torment, tension, sleep deprivation, sensory system, hearing, irritation, pituitary, instinct, otherworldliness, creativity, in arranging and keeping your mind calm.

9. Emerald: Related to lymph, labor, development, respiratory system, blood, heart, adjusting glucose, monogamy, love, trustworthiness, a sleeping disorder, harmony, expelling sadness, and so forth.

10. Malachite: Related to the liver, respiratory system, kidney stones, vision, aggravation, outrage, fixation, insight, and circulatory system.

11. Sapphire: fevers, hearing issues, consume, T.B, instinct, mental clearness, lessening irritation, nosebleeds, and communication.

12. Ruby: Related to cholesterol, blood purifying, love, boldness, stamina, blood clusters, authority, feelings, contaminations, impotence, and imperativeness.

13. Rose Quartz: Related to cherish, tranquility, excellence, pardoning, benevolence, outrage, enthusiastic equalization, and so on.

Types of Crystals and How to Use

Precious stones come in such vast numbers of changing shapes, hues, and sizes that frequently it tends to confound choosing which one to utilize or wear, particularly when you don't know about the chakra framework or of the atmosphere. It would take a book to cover each precious stone in detail, yet I have recorded only a couple of the most well-known gems and their employments.

Rose Quartz: This precious stone is pink in shading. A bit of rose quartz is perfect in the home on a table or seat top, mainly where some hyperactive youngsters or individuals have an excess of energy. The beautiful shading pink mitigates and mends, particularly when an individual has misfortune or disturbed in their life. Wearing a rose quartz gem brings harmony where there is disharmony and help in improving a messed up heart.

Smokey Quartz: This is a ground-breaking and profound stone. It is an establishing stone as it can ground overabundance energy. It is for contemplation and is an exceptionally fantastic healer.

Amethyst: The amethyst is a genuinely otherworldly stone. It is an incredibly ground-breaking emotional balancer and a trustworthy healer. It has been said that amethyst is the stone for individuals who have addictions. It is a brilliant stone to have along the edge of the bed to enable you to rest and magnificent for anybody with a cerebral pain. I have realized individuals dependent on resting pills, which gave them away once they found how the amethyst could assist them with sleeping.

Clear Quartz: This gem is an incredibly fantastic healer. It deals with all parts of the psyche and body and is extremely powerful for giving you certainty and for expelling antagonism. It can build your standard energy stream just as work on all parts of the auric body. Individuals who have abundant energy, however, may locate that wearing a reasonable, quartz gem can make them significantly increasingly hyperactive. For these individuals, a masterpiece of an alternate shading would likely be better.

Tiger's Eye: Tiger's eye can be an earthy red, blue, or dark-colored. However, the majority of the tiger's eye gems are establishing stones, implying that they can ingest overabundance energy. Regularly when I get a development of mental power, I hold two tiger's eye tumble stones, one in each hand, and can feel the abundance of energy from my body filling the rocks. When I need strength, I can generally hold the stones again and ingest energy from them. They additionally are relieving to take a gander at and are glorious for hyperactive youngsters.

Just as being worn, precious stones can be utilized to enable you to contemplate. The best sort of precious stone for this is a little group of plain quartz or a massive bit of quartz. I find that holding the precious stone in the left hand is perfect for reflection; however, a few people lean toward the right side. It truly is the thing that you feel best with. Intuition is the thing that you ought to consistently pursue concerning precious stones. When you believe you need to hold a specific precious stone, at that point, do as such. If a precious stone does not interest you and somebody says it is for you, don't acknowledge it. Continuously pursue your senses, and you won't turn out badly.

Chapter 7: Stones And Their Healing Properties

AGATE This stone is used to strengthen the heart and to give courage. In Brazil it is recognized that Agate decreases the fever and even has the same characteristics as soothing pure water. It is also used to sharpen the vision, to lighten the mind, to make eloquence and to seek gold. The mossy agate increases strength. Amulets are also useful in insanity and mental illness. This stone has been said to increase the strength of its holder's moon, boost his self-esteem and sexual appetite.

AQUAMARINE The stone of the clarificators, the mystics of the pure soul, can experience all of the clarity of the mental vision and its omniscience. It was used for the eyes. It is best to use close to the heart so that it can affect the solar plexus. This protects combat nerve pain, organ dysfunction, disorders in the chest, chin and mouth, and teeth, toxins and stomach pain. It protects our employees.

Dark-green ALEXANDRITE type. It was said to expose the lies and errors of people near us. The name comes from Czar Alexander II. It was useful for the nervous system and prevents different types of cancer.

AMAZONITE It helps improve speech of the body. It has been said to promote and sooth the brain and nervous system. The heart and the physical body are improved. It assists in the delivery of births. This emphasizes male qualities. Great for whom artistic practices are involved.

AMBER It is a fossilized pine tree liquid extract that existed millions of years ago. Small bugs, flowers and seeds from the prehistoric period are contained in this resin. Amber is said to have the power to repel body diseases. It is helpful to place a part of the body that is unbalanced or painful. This releases the negative energy and allows the body to heal. It is also prescribed for suicidal people or people with a destructive propensity.

AMETHYST It is the third eye sign that sees everything. It was said to alleviate sadness, resentment and depression. When the mind is in an oppressed state, it has a calming effect. It is also the rock for social resolutions. This helps with sleeplessness.

This stone and its radiant dark blue tone helped to change towards conscious thinking, to purify the mind and soul. It was also stated, it activates the highest thinking, enriching the soul. It can be extended to every part of the body that is blocked physically.

BLACK ONYX Mineral was used to help alleviate the issue. It was used to position the great pyramid in the king's chamber. It was used to promote awesome truths and memories that rise to the surface of the conscious mind.

The strength of our mental power is favoured by CALCITE. It is the rock of our lymphatic system, and our renal activity has been said to support.

The energy is close to the sun: it warms and gives life. CITRINE or YELLOW QUARTZ. It can draw wealth related to physical and material energy. She said she was helpful for problems like poor digestion, renal infection and bladder, constipation and other stomach problems. It is the most suitable for earthly matters, interpersonal relations or familiar matters.

CORAL It's been used around the neck for anemia and body fatigue. It can combat jealousy and helps in the event of infertility. For a harmonic relationship with nature, its use is often suggested.

CORALINE Good for unfocused and distracted. It was mentioned that it helps the mind to stay right now. And in cases of impotence and sexual vulnerability it can be useful. For the citizens with shyness and courage, it is used to improve their voice and self-confidence.

CRISOCOLA It is a feminine stone reflecting the passive and emotional water and the sun. It is said to be suitable for typical female issues, such as nausea, lower back pain, anxiety and birth function. This encourages emotional balance, alleviates sorrow and anger and trades these feelings for forgiveness and understanding.

CRISOPASIO or CHALCEDONY Sexuality was declared to stimulate. The stone was also composed for the sexual organs and used for sexual diseases. Great with issues with eyesight.

The pure white light emitted by it includes all colors, which makes it regenerative and energizing. It is great for recovery sessions. It has a very strong radiant aura, recommended for harmonizing the atmosphere. It is the stone of spiritual wisdom and farsightedness.

Diamond It is stated to improve brain functions. Diamond This removes the barriers in CHAKRA coronary and personality. This is a great healer. This is a great healer. This eliminates the anger. The external and ethereal body is cleaned. It represents the spiritual dimensions of will and power. This purifies and purifies. This increases physical strength and courage.

Diopsidio It is the stone used for the realization of great projects and the success of businesses. It has been found effective for digestive system diseases.

Dolomite Calcium and magnesium rich in this rock. It was written for the use of the bones and growth of the skeleton and the muscles. Good for those who have weak teeth or cavities.

Emerald It has said that it helps to develop a good body and revitalize the physical body after severe illness. This normalizes the tension of the artery. It was used for infection of the eye. Its continuous use encourages the acquisition of wealth and assets.

Enxofre Originated from volcanoes and helps treat breathing conditions like asthma, pneumonia, sore throat, etc. It is used to purify the body from harmful toxins and to protect the joint.

Fluorite It is used to counter any kind of mental disorder, which allows the consciousness to grow. It is useful for arranging ideas and avoiding excessive distraction.

Galena The strong carrier of mental sensations and supernatural phenomena, such as telepathy, etc, Goethite It supports a blood-weak and asthma-driven circulatory system. It is also recommended for the diagnosis of nervous frailty and general body fatigue. It injects good humor and vitality and enhances the character.

Granite Useful for different hormonal malfunctions or infections, spy for sexual organs (venereal diseases). Granite. It is recommended to wear next to the body, because it energizes the mind and gives the person beauty and joy.

It's a good cold weather stone when people feel cold and have little energy. Its most common use was to stop hemorrhages. It gives courage, calms nerves and wipes away cold.

Jade This stone stimulates psychical concentration and development. It helps to achieve a high degree of mysticism and reveals dark personality aspects.

Jasper It has always been related to magical, strong and healing properties. It was used in the bowel button to avoid stomach injury.

Kunzite It's a good stone near the heart. The goal is to prepare self-esteem for everlasting expressiveness. It can balance the brain with the soul. It was told to soothe the frustration, nervousness and fear.

It is the rock of reflection and meditation. Lapis Lazuli. It has excellent purification properties. It attracts the mind inside to find its power source.

Petrified Wood The blood toner is said to be. It helps to create a successful animated state during daytime activities. It was said that when applied against mental fatigue it was better.

Malachite Power consumed. When applied to sick or painful areas, energy can be extracted and psycho-emotional causes that cause distress are established. May help release the diaphragm pressure and restore a deep respiration.

Olivina has enabled the digestive system to prevent inflammation and infection, such as cramps, ulcers, and irritability, after an extremely busy time of work.

Onyx It refers to the earth, the physical, the survival and the fulfillment of the personal ego. It was said that it functions as a magnet and draws supernatural powers to the body. Its use is perfect for airmen or those who lean towards fantasy exaggeration. It is a foundation that helps solve financial problems.

Opal It has been said that it helps children to develop and fosters feelings of goodness and friendship. It is a gem of goodness, devotion, imagination and faith. Heat, flame and ether are there. It must be held in a chain of gold or a circle of gold.

Moonstone It absorbs the moon's power, calms the mind and is linked to human emotions. It was used to relieve stress and depression. It is useful for defending against disruptive patterns. It helps men to attract the female.

Cross Stone It is known as the stone of mysticism and of faith that move mountains since ancient times. The pilgrims took it on their religious journeys, as it led them and protected them from danger and tentation. In this rock, the cross-design represents the four cardinal points and the faith itself. It is by far the stone of happiness that attracts money, love and energy. It protects against aggression and risk.

Pyrite It was noted that it was effective for the treatment of respiratory problems applied to the mouth. This helps to relieve bronchitis and allergies. It is called the stone that attracts wealth and money because of its resemblance to gold, which contributes to good business transactions.

Blue Quartz Patience, sensitivity and empathy are to be created. The anti-inflammatory sedative has been noted and it controls hormones. It is effective against menstrual pain. It encourages relationships and communication and stimulates spontaneous and casual behavior.

Rose Quartz The soothing and calming rose color of this rock is used to alleviate accumulated heart sorrows. IT dissolves the accumulated cargo that suppresses the ability to love. This emanates energy that replaces sorrow, anxiety and anger, and is said to overcome emotional problems.

It has been noted that it improves the nutrition, enhances blood circulation and restores the energies of the skin. Green Quartz and Aventurine It was told to give love and games luck.

It has been said that it soothes and calms the heart. Rhodocrosite It has also been noted that it has a major influence on the creative process, the subconscious mind and prevents depression. This induces good feelings in the human heart.

Ruby Concentration has been said to support and gives mental strength. It was noted, it reinforces the heart. This should be used in the left hand with gold. It served for flow of the blood.

Sapphire This worked against adverse effects. This supports rheumatics, aches, seizures and anxiety in the nervous system. It encourages deep relaxation and prayer.

Princess Blue Sodalite It was said that it reinforces creative communication and expression. It helps to be straighter and less critical of existence. It helps to look at the goals after they are met. It was noted that it encourages bravery and endurance.

Topaz It is noted that it encourages enthusiasm and alleviates fear. It was said that it gives strength and intelligence. Topaz has indoor magnetized. This encourages clarity of mind. The ethereal glow encourages the joy of life and the power of seeing life in the future optimistically. It is best to put it into a pocket in times of doubt and uncertainty. It helped to make the right decisions.

Blue Turmaline The good function of the lungs and throat was noted. It helped with insomnia and makes sleep calm and restful.

Black Tourmaline It said negative energy should be repelled. You tell, it's security.

It has been noted that it can absorb harmful stimuli that can take over its bearer. When the holder's ill, the color changes. It protects against pollution of the environment. It is considered sacred to the Buddhists of Tibet.

Reiki Healing Hands

What are the Reiki Healing Hands?

Healing hands could be the term offered to people who have been attuned to the healing power of Reiki Healing and can perform Reiki's channeling of this power through their hands.

What does Reiki mean?

Reiki is typically a type of soothing hand, whose roots date back thousands of years to Christ and Buddha in India and the East. Usui Reiki is a reiki strategy developed in the 19th century by Dr Mikao Usui. Usui created the name REIKI himself, Rei which means Life Force, Universal and Ki. Usui developed this reiki system to ensure that anyone can practice healing. He wanted Reiki to be universal, so that regardless of religious or cultural background you had, you could become a master of reiki. Both adults and children can use Usui Reiki.

Reiki can be a gift of life and self preservation that is reflected in the genetic composition of all creatures of Gods. It is the higher connection with divine force that brings life into all the living tissues. It is with omniscient understanding that we are all born to cure and preserve life, with all living things unified by the universal life force, the non-physical omnipresent power that gives life to every living organism.

How could you get Reiki?

Reiki from a licensed Reiki practitioner can be received. You can also do Reiki on your own by Reiki. We agree that the Essence Of Reiki home study course would be the best home study course to learn about Reiki, we used this course and we found it extremely simple and enjoyable. You may be a licensed Usui Reiki Master or Pet Reiki Master immediately after the course is completed.

Reiki Healing Reiki will help you improve any aspect of your life and help you maintain good health and prevent diseases. It's for everyone and can be used for healthy adults, young people, infants, unborn young people and animals as well. It is a safe and easy choice for counseling to support and improve the effects of routine treatment for a person in the hospital or wellness centre. Reiki is used in a wide range of settings, including hospitals, hospitals, support groups for cancer, post-operative recovery and drug rehabilitation. Reiki may also be used with other natural healing therapies, including meditation, crystals and aroma therapy, with Reiki strengthening the effect of such treatments.

We have received and conducted Reiki on numerous occasions as Usui Reiki Masters. We truly feel that Reiki's healing power is an extraordinary thing and afterwards we feel extremely relaxed. The most effective way to fully understand what healing hands are or feel is to observe them for the place of your self-reiki hand. So soon as you receive your very first degree, a Reiki Master will make you willing to work with the common power of life. Nonetheless, you must know that with every discipline, there is a first training and mastering of the healing techniques, including the required Reiki Hand positions, to achieve Reiki Self Therapy. Mrs. Takata advises her students first to heal themselves, then their parents, then their good friends. Only then did she think she would be adequately trained and able to work as a doctor and cure others.

Learning the Reiki hand positions can be compared to learning when someone first learns to drive an automobile, they require time, practice and experience to understand what seems to be a complex set of techniques. Nonetheless, within a very short space of time they can drive safely and easily as they instinctively control the car and all the other driving skills.

Also, you can learn the skills and techniques relevant to Reiki healing art, such as reiki hand positions, with time, practice and experience. Treat the early months like an apprenticeship as an insight into the situation; this can give you time to build confidence and experience. Because the more you practice with Reiki, the more intuitive you will be, the stronger the energy frequency will probably be and a new positive balance will be established and felt in your life.

Using the Reiki hand positions when carrying out a self-healing reiki could be the foundation for individual development and self-discovery. Reiki will not only be a healing tool; it will also offer security, preventance and private transformation at all stages. As you progress along the new path, you will inevitably encounter obstacles and setbacks in your life that usually appear as the entire seaside, but in Reiki you will have the strength to cope like pebbles on the beach. Even if you do not use Reiki to cure anyone other than yourself, you will experience a brand new sense of equilibrium and harmony in your life.

No other self-treatment process is as quick and effective as Reiki. Just because Reiki is generally available to you, if you feel tired, depressed and have any pain or ache, all you can dois lay your hands across your body. Reiki's infinite wisdom will go wherever it is necessary.

Recharge the battery every day, not only when challenges, problems, anxieties or illnesses occur. Day-to-day self-remedy will help prevent infection and illness, and easily concentrate and stabilize your life. Whenever you use Reiki on yourself, you enhance your self appreciation and adoration. You will discover and grow your mission in life into further compassion and love.

You get into touch with every day, including traffic jams, instead of being overwhelmed in normal actions; conferences, interviews, go to the doctor?Dental practitioner waiting at the queues, your young people need to name but a few and your family's commitments allow Reiki to enter your life and make Reiki a brand new way of life for you.

Reiki is a pleasure to taste and to appreciate. Keep in mind the more Reiki you use, the stronger and deeper it gets. Every day, your personal life could be extended by a few years.

You will consider some positive aspects to benefit which take place without effort from a Reiki self-treatment like: Reiki can help you if you're depressed. Reiki centering your mind if you're uncertain Reiki powers, if you're feeling exhausted Reiki calms you down after you're scared. When you absorb all of Reiki's power much more intuitively, you can transfer your hands to wherever you feel right. Having said that, if you know of a particular problem like injury or pain, you must begin by putting your hands directly across that region and follow-up with complete self-treatment.

At the outset, a set procedure with the chakra points is often best followed.

You can leave every self-treatment to your intuition after you have mastered the hand positions. You may want to work with music to create the right mood. Find a spot where, if possible, you won't be interrupted. You will normally spend between three and five minutes on each role.

Nonetheless, time is usually short, but note that a little Reiki is better than no Reiki. A large glass of purified water is drank during self therapy. Close your eyes and go in and be mindful of the thoughts and emotions that emerged during the session. You can feel light headed, and this is for those who have to rest and sit down to get a short time.

Astrology of the Chakras

Many of us are now well aware that the "human energy field" consists of seven main energy centers or chakras clustered along the brain-spinal axis. Each core is acting as a substation or conduit of universal or prana energy flowing through the medulla at the base of the skull. As the prana goes down through the lower five chakras, it is changed and altered by its pure state. If the lower chakras are clear and free from adverse experiences (trauma, repression, etc.) the prana is free to climb back into the upper chakras leading into higher consciousness levels.

If however the lower chakras are blocked, the prana is blocked, and these energetic obstructions start to appear as cognitive, emotional and physical "discontinuation." In other words, if we have blockages in any of the chakras it means that we have broken our attenuation at a subtle or not so sutil level with the universal life force energy. Since the chakras are energy centers that respond to vibration, one way we can return to harmonization or harmonization is by actively using rhythm, music and movement.

One of the tools that can help us on this path is to understand the relationship between chakras and planets through the use of astrology. Each chakra is related or ruled by a different planet in the astrological universe. The astrological map at the energetic level shows not only the position of the planets but also the interrelation and the state of the chakras. Essentially, we have our inner solar system that directs our consciousness ' development into different centers of the chakra. By understanding the planetary qualities of each chakra, we can use specific forms of music, vibration and movement to open and energize each chakra.

Chakras Astrology The first chakra at the base of the spine is linked to planet Saturn. Astrologically, Saturn reflects our desire to anchor ourselves and make our dreams come true. In our lives, not enough Saturn leaves us underground and unable to support us. For some, it is difficult for Saturn to create a sense of strong boundaries and a centre. Nevertheless, we can keep too much of Saturn and resist changes on the material plane because of insecurity and fear. One way to heal the first chakra is by linking to the earth's energies. Walking barfoot, yoga and drumming are all ways of tapping into the first chakra's low frequencies. In general, drumming is an active way to open and awaken the first chakra. When we dance, we always hold the drum between our feet, which connects directly to the first chakra on the base of the spine. Through tuning the lower frequencies of the drum we not only become energized but also more present and alive in our bodies.

The other chakra, ruled by Jupiter, is found in the body's pelvic and genital region. The second chakra has to do with imagination and sexuality and how we can transfer energy and feelings to our fundamental vital forces. Jupiter is the planet, astrologically, which shows how we expand our consciousness. If we grew up in a family that suppressed emotions or sexuality, it directly affects the second chakra and the sense of expansion. When one region in the second chakra is blocked, sexuality is said, then all the other areas are affected: desire, imagination, expression of deep emotion. We are in contact with our innate life force or kundalini power when the second chakra is open. This is our fundamental electrical force, which animates our bodies and, once freely articulated, produces magnetism, excitement and genuine creativity.

The key to the energy of the second chakra is to transmit, open and extend our instinctual capacity. One of the best ways I can do this is through free form or African dance. Any movements that expand the region of the second chakra or pelvis may lead to this core's energy loosening. We are also excellent with the use of ethnic or world music, which stimulate the instinctual or moving core, like didgeridoos.

The power is based on the third chakra that is located on the solar plexus or hara. Mars, the individual will of the world and Pluto, the common will of the universe. The problems of the 3rd chakra are linked to strength, order, trust and empowerment of one's intestines. A blocked third chakra could be lack of decision-making, a lack of trust in our instincts and a sense of oppression and aggression. A third overactive chakra may be a question of power, stalking, rage or violence. The principal cure for the third chakra, without injuring others, is to learn how to gain power. You must also learn how to overcome the feeling that you are out of reach.

Music can be a particularly powerful tool for opening the third chakra, since it is a nonverbal interaction that circumvents the conscious mind and directly reaches our deepest emotions. Many people who think their emotions must be controlled are separated by evocative songs. Anything that moves you either emotionally or physically is a way to become deeper, often caught up in the third chakra, emotions of anger, sorrow and rage. The third chakra will grow when those emotions are noticeable and expressed and the energy can now become more rewarding forms of self-presentation and creativity.

The 4th chakra is regulated around the heart and lungs by the planet Venus. Venus is what we admire, how we love and how we can express our love unconditionally. I always attribute the "higher" governance of the fourth chakra to Planet Neptune as Neptune serves a cycle that transcends our individuality and union with spirit and divine love.

The fourth chakra is the bridge of the lower chakra with the middle. Our western culture mainly concerns money, gender and power in the first three chakras. When we clear up the emotional relation between the first three chakras, the vast qualities of the higher chakras can then be explored. When we block the fourth chakra, we might be afraid not to be accepted, to give and receive affection or non-fulfillment.

The heart chakra is restored through the development of love, devotion and connection to others. Music can open the heart and in the case of devotional singing, minimize feelings of separation. Samuel Lewis ' Sufi style dances of mutual peace are an ideal way to combine sound and acts in order to facilitate spiritual relations and unity with others. Universal Peace Dances combine sacred mantras from various spiritual traditions with basic circle dances, which help us break the imaginary barriers that hold us apart. They are also a very safe way to give and receive love without any constraints.

Mercury, the planet of all forms of communication, and Chiron, which represents the mentor / teacher archetype, regulate the fifth chakra in the gargot region. The fifth chakra helps us to express ourselves and to make our life. We can be afraid to say or talk to one another if the fifth chakra is blocked. The desires or thoughts from the chakra of the heart may also be difficult to express. Another shared manifesto of a blocked fifth chakra is the unbelief in our ability to create our life as we wish. We have finally stopped trusting in the power of our free will, if we have grown up without any say, or have mocked our choices.

The fifth chakra must be healed if we are to open up the sixth and seventh chakra intuitive awareness. If the fifth chakra is blocked, we can't be too abstract and continuously channel the implicit intuitive knowledge through the higher centers. Singing is one of the best ways to open the 5th chakra as far as healing is concerned. Since many people "breaked" literally with 5th chakra blockages, the best way to reassert our identity is by toning! It is also helpful to choose sacred mantras, like OM, because OM is seen as the fundamental or primordial notation of the universe. When we sing OM, we remember the creative sound that all material types must make.

In the middle of the forehead the sixth chakra is co-ruled by the sun and moon, between the eyes. The sixth chakra is connected to our better mental ability to observe, assess, consider and appreciate oneself. Historically, the sixth chakra has two bars. The pole of the moon on the medulla has the "breath of heaven" and God's power. The third eye's sun or active poles convey this essential power through our personality. A blocked sixth chakra may be anxious to look at yourself, anxious to use your intuitive abilities, refused to learn about life experiences or inability to receive your inner guidance. Physical symptoms may include migraines, anxiety, depression and learning loss. Relaxation, creativity and dreamworking in the creative world are one of the best means to open the sixth chakra. Art, which evokes imagination and opens us to the world of unexpected insights, may encourage this opening. In particular, several CDs are available to help the brain enter the deeper consciousness of the alpha, delta and theta which is only generated through meditation otherwise.

At last we hit the seventh chakra on top of the head or crown. The chakra of the Crown is known as another energy input of life force and shapes our connection to the universal consciousness. I associate the seventh chakra with the planet Uranus as Uranus is the universal flow of energy which nourishes mind, body and spirit. Uranus is the kundalini force at the base of the spine on the first chakra from Vedic point of view in India. As a consequence of each chakra, kundalini energies increase the backbone and activate the seventh chakra, resulting in enlightenment or illumination. There are many experiencing this in orgasm when the kundalini reaches the lower chakras and activates the chakra. It is not usually that we channel so much energy into higher centres, so that we avoid or become unaware that we are going to sleep after orgasm.

If the 7th chakra blocks it may be conveyed as low vital energy, a world doubt, or a sense of meaning or direction in our lives. The only way to open it up or down is the Seventh Chakra, the polar side to the first Chakra. Pranayama or breathing practices help the seventh to increase our body's capacity to transmit energy. If we expand our channeling capacity, then we can deal with more resilience across our bodies without resistance.

As we move and listen to the lower chakras, we lower the pressure and release latent energy at the base of the spine. That is, opening up the higher chakras is not to suggest that we should neglect or "transcend" the lower chakras, as some traditions would have us believe. Alternatively, we must strive to open up the whole area of the chakra in a grounded and personalized way to perceive higher conditions.

Chapter 8: Your Own Collection

Now that you understand how crystals work and how to use them properly, it's time to start building your own private, and very personal, collection of healing crystals. This entails a little more than just walking into the first store you see and buying whatever takes your fancy. Buying crystals takes time, attention and careful consideration. This entire chapter is dedicated to helping you choose the right crystals and to teach you how to take care of them.

Choosing the Right Crystals

The first thing you need to do when buying a crystal is to decide what you want it to do. Buying a crystal with a specific purpose in mind is a much better idea than simply choosing a crystal for the sake of owning one. You have an idea of which types of crystal have the right abilities, so keeping your mind focused on what you want to do with the crystal, walk through the store and let your intuition choose for you. Don't think about it. Feel it. A specific crystal might catch your eye for no specific reason, or you might feel one of the crystals pulling at you. That is a good indication that that is the crystal for you. Hold the crystal in your hand and focus your energy on it. You should feel something from it, like sensations of hot or cold, pulsations, or simply just a sense of rightness. If this is the case, you've found your crystal. If you don't feel anything from the crystal you've selected, your search continues. Spotting a crystal through this sense can be difficult at first, but it becomes easier with practice. Sometimes it's simply the color of the crystal or an interesting shape that draws your attention, and that's okay. The crystal chooses you as much as you choose it. Just listen to your instincts and you shouldn't have a problem. Beyond crystals won't work for you, there are even crystals that will work against you. There is nothing wrong with you or the crystal. It just means that the energy in your body vibrates at a frequency that clashes with that of the crystal. Owning a crystal like this can have a very negative influence on your crystal healing process, but a simple way to see if a crystal will reject you is to close your hand around the crystal and hold it against your stomach. Close your eyes and focus on the crystal. You'll definitely feel the crystal pushing against you, trying to get away from your energy. In many cases, you can even see the crystal pushing your body away slightly if the clash is strong enough.

Basic Crystals for Beginners

If you're a beginner, it can be very difficult to know which crystal to buy, especially if you're trying crystal healing out for the first time and you don't have any idea about what to expect or what you want to do with your crystals. Crystal healing might not be for you, and you don't want to end up spending a fortune on a large variety of crystals to experiment with in the hopes that one or two might work for you. To prevent that, here is a list of a few simple, strong crystals that are easy to come by, inexpensive, and bound to tell you if crystal healing is meant for you.

• Clear quartz, which amplifies the effects of your other crystals and amplifies your intention. It is often called the *Master Healer* because it can be used for almost any purpose.

• Amethyst, which is a strong spiritual stone and can be used as a stress reliever or to help in your meditation. Amethyst is a great crystal to have with you in difficult times when you need to look deep into yourself for answers, or when you need an emotional and spiritual boost.

• Tiger's eye carries strong earth energies, making it great for grounding yourself and helping you make logical decisions. It also channels creative energy and can help you get rid of writer's block.

• Bloodstone is a crystal that helps boost the immune system, boosts energy, causes relief for chronic diseases and clears the body of disease and toxins. This stone is well known as the healing crystal, and it's a great aid for athletes.

• Carnelian encourages confidence and motivation. It also awakens passion and attractions and can be used to enhance your sexual experience.

• Smoky quartz is another earth stone that grounds you. It is also great for cleansing your other crystals and the energy in a space, as it draws out negative energy quite well. Smoky quartz is good for relieving panic attacks, negative emotions, and negative memories.

• Hematite is a good barrier stone that provides mental and emotional stability. It encourages blood circulation and draws toxic energy out of your body. Because hematite assists memory function and gives you mental clarity, it's a good stone to keep around when studying.

Where to Buy Crystals

Finding the right place to buy your crystals takes a little homework. Not all stores sell crystals, and specialized crystal stores that sell a large variety and can properly cater to your needs are much less common than we would like. Furthermore, not all stores that sell crystals can be trusted. Many jewelry stores and pharmacies will sell crystal jewelry and birthstones that look authentic enough at first glance but are as often as not nothing more than colored glass. This isn't necessarily an evil plot to sucker you out of your money, but simply a good way to sell more items meant as decorations rather than healing tools. Any healing effects gained from these crystals are a result of the placebo effect, where your mind convinces your body that the crystals are working. Not all of these types of crystals are necessarily fake, mind you, and if you can verify that they are the real deal, you can buy as many of these crystals as you want.

The best place to buy crystals is at a store that specializes in selling them. Because crystals for the purpose of crystal healing aren't a global franchise, these stores tend to be small and tucked into odd corners of the world. These stores can even be businesses run out of the owner's home. In any case, the chances of finding a specialized store in your local mall aren't all that big. Do some research to find a crystal shop in your area, and see if there are any reviews on the place before you take the trip. If you're just moving around town, it won't be hard to recognize one of these stores. A good trademark is a display window filled with crystals of all shapes and sizes, ranging from small carved figures to clusters of raw crystals large enough to cover your hand. Even if they are perfectly organized, shops like these tend to have an organic, natural feel to them, and if you've ever worked with crystal healing before, you should be able to feel something of the energy of the crystals the second you pass through the door.

Shopping online is also a viable option, especially if you don't have a crystal store in your area. Online suppliers often have a very large variety, and it's possible to see what they can get their hands on for you, even if they don't have the supplies on hand. Again, shopping at sites that specialise in crystals and related products is better than general places that sell a bit of everything. Still, a word of caution: not all websites out there are trustworthy. Be careful where you give out your personal information, and don't jump the gun on this one. Do your homework on the sites you visit, and make sure they aren't trying to scam you. Just by scrolling through a few of their pages can easily tell you if they know what they're talking about, and if a site is popular with a lot of frequent customers, it's a good sign that it is trustworthy and provides good services and products. Reading as many reviews given to these websites as possible is also a good way to learn what you can expect from them. The biggest setback of shopping online is that you can't be there to choose your crystal in person and feel its energy. This makes finding the ideal crystal for you harder, but you can still go far with this form of shopping.

How to Spot a Fake

If you're at all interested in crystal healing it is critical that you know the difference between a real and a fake crystal. Fake crystals can do a great deal for you if you just want a nice piece of jewelry or a decoration for your home, but no matter how beautiful they are, these cut and colored piece of glass, resin or plastic have no helpful energy or healing properties. Another type of fake is when your cheaper, more common types of crystals are dyed to resemble rarer and more expensive crystals. The surest way to detect if a crystal is a fake or not is through a series of scientific tests, but trying to do that in a store is a little ridiculous. Here are some simple tips for discovering a fake on sight.

- To detect the difference between clear quartz and glass or resin, look for bubbles. Real quartz crystals may have flaws inside, but they do not have small, perfectly round bubbles.

- Look for flaws. Crystals are not perfect, and that is where their beauty lies. If a line in a crystal is too regular and the same thickness all around, they may be glass. If the color is too perfect and solid, it's most likely dyed. Transparent and translucent crystals have interesting little flaws on the inside that can be hard to recreate.

- With crystal points, look at the symmetry. If a crystal point is unusually symmetrical, it isn't natural. It was cut that way.

- Hold transparent and very translucent crystals against a piece of paper or card with some writing on it. Real crystals won't magnify the letters, and some may even blur the letters a little. Glass crystals tend to magnify letters.

- Check the color. If a crystal has an unnaturally bright, rich or neon color to it, it is likely that the crystals have been dyed or treated.

- Check the base of the crystal for paint or glue. It often happens that the base of a crystal is painted to make its color look richer, and crystal clusters might be a bunch of rocks glued together.

- Ask the seller. In some cases fake crystals aren't there because the seller wants to cheat you, but because they know some people just want something pretty. They will most likely be more than happy to tell you if there are any fake crystals or crystals that have been dyed.

- Check for extremely deep cracks. It often happens that small crystal chunks that normally aren't useable are ground into a fine powder. This powder is poured into a mold and compressed to form a new, larger crystal. These crystals tend to have deep cracks.

- Check for excess dye in the cracks of a crystal.

- Check the price. If a rare or normally expensive crystal us unexpectedly cheap, chances are it isn't real.

- Try to find out if the seller is a trustworthy supplier by asking around about them and looking them up. Reviews are a good way to find out more about the supplier.

- Know your crystals. Before buying crystals, do a bit of research on the crystals you are interested in buying to find out their typical colors, shape, rarity and price range. This can do a lot to help you detect some obvious fakes in a store.

These tips can help you a great deal, but some fakes are very well made, and many of these won't do you much good when you're shopping online, but there are some easy ways to test for a fake crystal at home.

• Give the crystals a good wash. In many cases, the dye on a crystal will wash right off.

• Press the tip of a hot needle against your crystal. This may not be very effective against glass, as it will react the same as real crystals, but it can help against other fakes. A real crystal will simply form a small scorch mark that you can remove easily enough, but plastic, resin, and compressed crystals will begin to melt.

• If the crystal is soft enough, make a small cut with a metal knife. Under a magnifying glass, a real crystal will have jagged edges around the cut while glass or resin will have smooth edges. You can also make a small cut to see if there is a different color under a layer of strong dye.

- With some crystals, like turquoise, you can use UV lighting to detect a fake or dyed crystal. It will take a little bit of research to find out which crystals will have a blacklight effect and which won't, but it's well worth the effort.

To help you look out for counterfeiting a little better, here is a list of crystals that are most commonly faked, dyed or treated:

- Agate
- Carnelian
- Citrine
- Clear quartz
- Lapis lazuli
- Purple and pink jade
- Smoky quartz
- Turquoise

There are some cases where crystals are treated or faked where it is a feature and not a dishonest practice. A good example Swiss blue- and London blue topaz, where a regular blue topaz is treated to give it these intense hues. Opalite is another good example. Opal is very rare in gem form and usually very expensive, but it is a very beautiful stone that plays with light and color in incredible ways. Opalite is a special type of glass that is treated to recreate these effects. Opalite can be cut and polished into various shapes and is popular as jewelry. In cases like these, it is a given that the crystals and gemstones are not natural, but many sellers will still explain this to you to make sure you understand. The prices of these crystals will also be made accordingly.

Something to consider is that while paying dearly for a turquoise, only to discover it's dyed howlite is unforgivable, not all fakes are necessarily bad. Compressed crystals may not be made of one solid rock, but they often still have the same healing properties if they aren't dyed to pose as more expensive crystals. Treated crystals may also do what you want them to do. As an example, citrine is a very rare crystal and it usually has a white wine or pale yellow color. In most cases, amethyst is treated with heat until it turns orange and is sold as citrine. This may not be too bad, as amethyst has properties and abilities very similar to citrine, and many people prefer the brighter, more vibrant stone in their jewelry. In this case, you have a fully functioning, beautifully colored crystal at a fraction of what you would normally pay for a real citrine. Dye isn't always too horrible either. Where is the harm in a blue lace agate that has had its color enhanced a little? The dye won't diminish its ability to heal. There are even synthetic crystals created in laboratories using the exact same methods and ingredients as their naturally grown counterparts, just a lot less time. These crystals are still basically the same thing. Even though it is very frustrating and disappointing when you buy a crystal, only to discover that it's a fake and you've been tricked out of your money, this isn't always the case with fake crystals. If the seller is open and honest with you about the fakes, you understand where you stand with these fakes and are still willing to pay a fair and reasonable price for what you get, there is no reason why you can't be satisfied with any of your crystals.

After Buying

Once you've bought your crystal, it's time to make it yours. The first thing you need to do is clear your crystal of all negative energy or the energy of everyone who touched the crystal before you. There are many different ways to cleanse a crystal, which will be discussed soon, and you should choose what works for you. You can then give your crystal a little more purpose by setting your intentions. This is often called *programming.* As mentioned above, it's better to buy a crystal with a purpose in mind, and programming is basically confirming that purpose with your crystal and filling it with your own energy and vibrations. This way it will be able to resonate better with you and give you the best results. Programming crystals isn't limiting your crystal to one purpose alone or telling it how to heal you, but telling it where you need its help the most. Like going to a doctor and telling them you have a sore throat. That way the doctor knows what to look for and where to start. Crystal programming is an option and not a necessity. It may be a good help for crystals you're carrying with you or using long term, you don't have to program a crystal if you don't feel it's necessary. If you want to, however, here is how it's done.

Find a quiet place where you won't be disturbed or interrupted.

Take your crystal in both hands and hold it at the same level as your third eye chakra.

Close your eyes, take a few deep breaths to find inner calm, focus on your crystal and your specific intention for it.

Either silently in your head or out loud, tell the crystal what you want it to do. You can ask however you're comfortable with, but some examples could help.

"I program this crystal to help me improve my relationship."

"I charge this crystal with the intention to strengthen my resolve and work ethic."

"Crystal, I ask you to help me by healing my aches and pains from this illness."

Again, it is important to do what works for you personally, and if you don't feel comfortable programming your crystal, you shouldn't force yourself to do it.

Caring for Your Collection

Like any healing implements, your healing crystals require care and maintenance to keep them working properly. No medical professional would dream of using a dirty scalpel or malfunctioning defibrillator. In the same way, you shouldn't use crystals that have lost their charge or are cluttered with unwanted and negative energy. There are three main parts to keeping your crystals at their best: cleaning, clearing, and charging.

Cleaning Crystals

No one likes a dirty crystal, and dust, grime and all manner of other forms of dirt can interfere with the energy of your crystal. Crystals that are used in direct contact with your body or to infuse water need to be cleaned very thoroughly to prevent harmful bacteria and diseases. For large display crystals, a frequent good dusting ought to be enough, but with carved crystals or crystal clusters, it will take a little more work to clean up the nooks and crannies that just love gathering dust. The simplest way to clean a crystal is by rinsing it off with water and washing it with a soft cloth. Unfortunately, some crystals like azurite, selenite, angelite, and phenakate will begin to dissolve in water, and they should be kept well away. In these cases, you should use a clean, dry cloth to rub the dirt away. When cleaning crystals, you should make sure your cloth is soft and won't shed any fibers. A good alternative is using an otherwise unused, soft-bristled toothbrush to clean your crystals. When handling your crystals, keep in mind how rough you are. Some crystals can take a bit of rough handling without any problems, but there are many types of crystals that are softer and tend to scratch or break if you aren't careful. You should be especially careful and gentle with crystal clusters that have small crystals connected to the grid by only a very small area.

Cleansing Crystals

This refers to clearing and cleaning the energy of your crystal and restoring it to its natural state. Crystals have a tendency to absorb energy from the world around them, including from other people. If people touch your crystals, it will automatically absorb their energy, which usually doesn't work well with your own. This could cause problems with the crystal's ability to resonate with your energy and heal you, and this is why you shouldn't have anyone else touching your crystals. Crystals will also absorb negative energy in the air that you don't want to be sent your way. Crystals used in healing sessions or to draw out and ward off negative energy are especially problematic in this regard. Crystals should be cleansed frequently to remove all this unwanted energy and make their energy pure and clean again. There are many different ways to cleanse a crystal. Some methods don't work well with certain types, and some can be more difficult to come by depending on time and place, but there are enough different methods for you to find something that works perfectly for you.

- Water is a great way to cleanse your crystals. Find a source of natural water like a pond, lake, river, spring or waterfall, and hold your crystal in the water for a while to let the clean water wash away the negative energy. You can even leave your crystal outside in the rain for a good cleansing. Leaving your crystal out a little longer during a thunderstorm can even help you charge your crystal with new energy. Of course, you shouldn't use this method on crystals that dissolve in water.

- Placing your crystals in saltwater for a few hours can also cleanse them, as the salt will help the water draw out and absorb the negative energy. Again, water isn't meant for all crystals, and you shouldn't use this method on crystals with a hardness lower than seven, as the salt can scratch and damage crystals that are too soft.

- The earth is a great cleanser, and you can harness this natural power by burying your crystals in the ground for about four hours or so. This is an especially strong method to use on earthy and grounding crystals like smoky quartz and tiger's eye. If you feel uncomfortable burying your crystal directly in the ground, you can place it in a glass container and bury the container. It isn't necessary for the entire container to be covered in earth.

• If you are fortunate enough to live in the right area, burying your crystal in clean, fresh snow is a great way to cleanse and charge your crystal.

• Natural light is also a good way to go. Sunlight has a very cleansing effect on your crystals and can burn away any unwanted energy if you leave your crystals outside for an hour or two on a bright sunny day. There are some crystals like amethyst, aquamarine, fluorite, citrine, rose, and smoky quartz that lose some of their color when exposed to direct sunlight, but luckily moonlight works too. Moonlight has the same cleansing effect as sunlight, but it will take a little longer.

The closer you are to a full moon, the stronger the effects. If you want to get an extremely thorough and potent cleansing and charging from the moon, you should put your crystals outside just after dusk and retrieve them shortly before dawn for twenty-eight consecutive days to expose the crystal to all the phases of a lunar cycle.

- Some crystals like clear quartz and carnelian have natural cleansing abilities, and you can use these to cleanse your other crystals. You can either place the crystal you want to cleanse on a larger cleansing crystal that will draw out the negative energy, or you could pack a circle of several small cleansing crystals around the crystal to be cleansed. These crystals may not need it as often as other types, but you shouldn't forget to cleanse your cleansing crystals every now and then too.

- Sage is a plant with many healing properties that can cleanse your crystal and restore its natural energy. To do this, set fire to some sage, it can be held in a bundle or loose in a fire-safe bowl, and move your crystal through the smoke of the sage. Thirty seconds of this should be enough, but if you feel the crystal needs a little more cleansing, add another thirty seconds. This process is called *smudging*, and should always be done outside or near a window.

• Probably one of the most simple and straightforward ways to cleanse a crystal is to leave it overnight in a bowl of brown rice. The brown rice will absorb all the negative and unwanted energy, and because of that, you shouldn't cook with it afterward. You can use the rice as compost, however.

• *Purple plates* or *positive energy plates* are devices sold at specialized stores and designed specifically to cleanse and charge your crystals. They are a great help but can be a little tricky to come by and tend to be slightly pricey. These plates aren't my first suggestion for beginners who are still just testing out the waters.

A good average to work by is cleansing your crystals about once a month, but you can never cleanse your crystals too often. A crystal in need of some cleansing will often feel slightly heavier, and you can feel its effects on you weakening. You'll also feel the presence of the negative energy within your crystals in severe cases. A cleansed crystal will feel lighter physically and in its energy. If you feel that a crystal is in need of cleansing, it doesn't matter how long ago you've cleansed it. You should cleanse it again. You should also cleanse your crystals before and after every meditation and healing session. If you're not carrying a crystal with you or have it placed in your home for a specific purpose, you should keep your crystals somewhere near windows and plants so they can constantly draw cleansing energy from nature and the sun and moon.

Charging Crystals

The same way people get tired at the end of the day and cellphone batteries die after a while, crystals will begin to lose their energy as they are used. There is only so much space for energy inside a crystal, and if it's used up completely, you will end up with a crystal that can barely do anything to heal or help you. This is a natural occurrence, and it is an easy solution to the problem: you simply need to charge the crystal with more energy. There various to charge crystals, and cleansing and charging can sometimes be done at the same time, using the same method. Here are some simple ways to charge your crystals:

● As with cleansing, you can expose your crystals to sunlight and moonlight for a few hours. Charging often takes longer than cleansing, and seven hours is a good general time frame, but how long you leave them exposed is up to you. It is important to make sure you don't expose the crystals to both sunlight and moonlight in the same charging session, as the two sources are quite different. If you're using sunlight to charge a crystal, exposing it to direct moonlight will change the energy in your crystal.

• Take your crystal to a place with a lot of nature, like a park or beach. Crystals can absorb positive, natural energy from the nature around them.

• Charge the crystal with some of your own energy. By keeping your crystal on you and focusing on sending your energy to the crystal, you can recharge the crystal using your own positive thoughts and energy.

• Again, just like with cleansing, water can be a great tool in recharging your crystals. Especially if you're using natural water or saltwater. The same goes for burying your grounding crystals in the earth.

• Fire is a great element for charging crystals. You can either do this by waving your crystal over a candle for a minute or so or by putting your crystals next to a fire for a short while. Be careful which crystals you use this method on and how long you leave them by the fire, as some types, such as amethyst, will change or lose their color if they are exposed to very high temperatures for too long.

- If you are willing to invest the money, purple plates and positive energy plates are designed to charge crystals as well as cleanse them.

- Smudging your crystals with sage will charge your crystals at the same rate that it will cleanse them.

- Crystals used for cleansing other crystals usually have a charging effect as well, and crystals that promote energy and physical activity can be very effective in giving energy to other crystals.

There is no set of rules for how frequently your crystals will need to be charged, and it is up to you to figure out what works for you. You should be able to feel if a crystal needs to be charged by the amount of energy you feel from it and how strongly it affects you when you're using it to heal, and you should charge your crystals whenever you feel they need it. In many cases, when you should charge a crystal depends on the crystal itself and how often you use them. Larger crystals tend to hold more energy than smaller ones, and some cuts and shapes are good for manifesting energy. These crystals don't need to be charged as often, but smaller crystals will lose their energy much faster. Crystals that are used frequently, such as those used for meditation, chakra aligning and healing sessions, will lose energy at a faster rate than those placed in rooms to gently radiate energy, and so should be charged more frequently. It's a good idea to charge these crystals before and after every time you use them. Crystal jewelry you wear constantly or crystals that you always keep in your purse or pocket will be the ones that need the most charging.

Luckily it is also very easy to charge them with your own energy, which you can do while you go through your day, or quickly taking a detour to your nearest park or sitting in your garden with your crystals a while.

Crystals can be an important tool in improving your life and health, and cleaning, cleansing and charging them should become second nature to you if you want to use them to their best potential. By neglecting to care for your crystals properly, you rob them of their ability to heal and reduce them to nothing more than pretty decorations and interesting jewelry.

Chapter 9: Diamond

Otherwise known as the Crystal of Light or the King of Stones, Diamonds are without a doubt the world's best known and most popular gemstone. Diamond has strong connections to winter and as a winter stone with its ice-like colour and clarity, it has a higher energetic frequency than usual, which may explain why it is the hardest mineral on Earth. In ancient Greece, Diamond was called *Adamas,* a word that means 'indestructible' or 'invincible' depending on the translation. Diamond is a 'master healer' capable of curing most common ailments as well as reducing stress, combatting exhaustion and clearing any energetic or emotional blockages affecting the Crown Chakra. In modern times Diamond is popularly associated with engagement and marriage and is said to instil loyalty, truth, trust and purity into a relationship. In older times Diamonds were worn by warriors due to the belief that the invisibility of the stone would enhance the natural abilities of the warrior rendering them impervious to attack whilst simultaneously bolstering the user's courage and strength in order to be victorious. Further to the pure energy radiated by Diamonds, they are also powerful amplifiers of energy and emotions, but beware, as Diamonds absorb both negative and positive emotions which if not cleansed can lead the wearer into less than satisfactory situations and emotional states. As a healer Diamond works as a 'support stone' supporting and aiding the medication/therapy or other treatments as well as the body's natural healing process. It is also said that Diamonds can cure all manner of conditions associated with purging the body of its waste and toxins, including constipation and water retention and may also enhance the wearer's cognitive abilities, nervous system and senses. Diamond is directly linked to the Crown Chakra but is also highly valued for its ability to activate, open, and balance all of the chakras, illuminating our inner-selves with its reflective energy, giving clarity, balance, and fortitude to overcome difficult situations. If your birthday falls under the star signs of Aries, Pisces or Scorpio it is advisable to avoid Diamond altogether as it is thought to have a negative effect on these signs bringing bad luck and disharmony to the wearer.

Colour

Clear

Birthstone

April

Zodiac

Virgo

Libra

Energetic Frequencies

Abundance

Money

Courage

Purity

Love

Chakras

The Crown Chakra

Activates all Chakras

Emerald

Emeralds have been revered by numerous cultures for thousands of years. They were worshipped by the Incans, were a symbol of everlasting life to the Egyptians, and have been traded in markets since at least the time of the Babylonians. Emerald is thought to enhance one's natural intuition by opening up the Heart Chakra and is sometimes known as the 'Stone of Successful Love'. Also referred to as the Travellers Protection Stone, Emerald is the perfect talisman for those travelling; its 'seeker energiser' energy aligns with and amplifies the Earth's natural energy to guide the wearer towards new experiences. Emeralds range from pale translucent green to deep vibrant greens and are truly some of the most beautiful crystals ever found. When used as a meditation tool, Emerald has the ability to lock in our rhythmic breathing patterns allowing for significantly deeper meditative states, promoting greater intuition, foresight and self-reflection. Emerald is a fantastic healing stone for those feeling exhausted or drained by filling the user with hope and encouragement, replenishing aura and strengthening the heart's energetic centre. The effect this has on the user helps those suffering from the loss of a loved one or the loss of one's own personal power or sense of safety. Emerald is also believed to speed up the healing process as well as vitalising and energising the lungs, liver, heart, and kidneys. Of all healing gemstones, Emerald is said to be the most efficient when it comes to healing the eyes and improving vision altogether. The purest of green rays emanate from the emerald and carry with them nature's wood energy and placing Emeralds in the family eating area of the home brings health, nourishment, and prosperity into the household.

Colour

Green

Birthstone

Aries

Gemini

Taurus

Zodiac

January

May

June

Planet

Venus

Energetic Frequencies

Love

Money

Protection

Chakras

The Heart or Fourth Chakra

Fluorite

Fluorite or the 'Stone of Positivity' for reasons unknown doesn't receive the attention of many of the more popular stones, however, this doesn't make it any the less beautiful or powerful. Fluorite forms in an array of colours and is known as the world's most colourful stone, the most common colour hues include shades of blue and purple, reds, oranges, browns, black, yellows and greens, and clear, and any combination of the above. The vast colour spectrum of Fluorite is due to the infinite combinations of mineral compositions that make up individual stones. Some of the rarer examples of Fluorite contain small amounts of extremely rare elements like cerium and europium leading to some stones possessing fluorescence, phosphorescence and on occasion thermoluminescent properties.

The dynamic energy carried by Fluorite clears and sharpens mental agility and heightens abilities related to manifestation, creativity, and magic. This is a powerful gemstone regularly used to reduce inflammation, cure cold and flu-like symptoms, stimulate the immune system and has antiviral and antibacterial properties. Emotionally, the differing colourings and types of Fluorite have unique meanings and properties specific to each individual stones mineral makeup, however, almost all types of Fluorite have a soothing and stabilising energy which settles erratic and imbalanced brainwave patterns and can make a huge difference to those suffering from mental illnesses and depression. Fluorite is the perfect gemstone for those feeling stressed or overwhelmed at work, its energy has the ability to promote coherent thoughts and clarity, situating one's conscious in the present moment by allowing past traumas to be forgotten and worries regarding the future to disappear. Ultimately, Fluorite is one of the most sought-after stones in the world and is respected by mineralogists, healers and spiritualists alike

Blue Fluorite

Used to purify the aura, specific areas or rooms, Blue Fluorite's vibrational frequency completely dissolves that of negative energy, organises scattered thoughts and when placed in the northernmost room in the house Fluorite's natural water energy calms and clears the atmosphere, creating the ideal are for study or prayer. When used as a meditation tool Blue Fluorite focuses the attention and relaxes the body making it possible to attain the state of 'no mind' which is essential for visions and spiritual journeys to the higher ethereal planes. Sometimes called 'The Healer of Souls' Blue Fluorite inspires honest communication and learning and its ability to negate stress and outside negativity makes it the perfect gemstone for those with a busy working life.

Green Fluorite

Green Fluorite's vivid yet pale colour hues regularly appear luminous to the eye and are without a doubt some of the most wonderful shades of green in the mineralogical world. Also called the 'Genius Stone' Green Fluorite is associated with learning and specifically attaining the highest levels of academic achievement. The vibrational energy of Green Fluorite stimulates both the left and right hemispheres of the brain, resulting in increased electrical activity within the brain leading to faster thought processing, inspired creativity, and a drastic increase in psychic ability. Green Fluorite is thought to help those suffering from addiction and heal both physical and emotional issues related to the heat through it energetic harmony with the Heart Chakra.

Yellow Fluorite

Yellow Fluorite is a crystal of unifying energy which inspires creativity and compassion, boosts intellect and resourcefulness and it has been claimed to even boost one's IQ. It is one of the best gemstones for focussing one's intent, providing mental clarity making the manifestation and realisation of ideas, ideals, and goals a significantly smoother process. Yellow Fluorite opens the Solar Plexus Chakra, having a balancing effect on the body's energetic network, bringing those affected feelings of support and resolution. When worn, Yellow Fluorite is great for healing skin complaints. It soothes ulcers, rashes, protects against infectious disease, and is particularly beneficial for those suffering from respiratory diseases.

Colour

Blue

Clear

Green

Purple

Yellow

Black

Brown

Multi-coloured

Birthstone

February (Blue)

March (Blue)

Zodiac

Pisces

Energetic Frequencies

Creation

Magic

Manifestation

Healing

Protective

Transformation

Chakras

The Throat Chakra (Blue)

The Brow Chakra (Blue, Yellow))

The Heart Chakra (Green)

The Solar Plexus Chakra (Yellow)

Chapter 6: Important Crystals, Their Uses, And Their Healing Powers

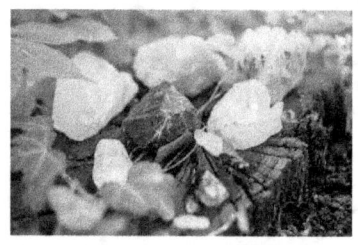

This and the next chapters are dedicated to giving you, a beginner in the realm of crystals, the top 25 stones and their amazing healing powers. It is time again to reiterate that crystals choose you and not the other way round. Therefore, read up about all the crystals mentioned in this book, choose one when investing for the first time, work with your chosen crystal for a while, and then make your subsequent choices.

Be patient with yourself and the crystal. Remember even human relationships take time and need to be nurtured to flourish. The same thing holds good for your relationships with crystals too. So, here goes a small list of crystals great for beginners to start working with.

Agate

Belonging to the quartz family, agate is a powerful healing crystal, thanks to the presence of silicon dioxide in it, an element that is also present in the human body. Known as a stabilizer, agate is the stone to call upon when you need grounding support and help during times of crisis. This crystal is abundantly found in many countries around the world.

The profile of agate has a dreamy quality about it as perfectly symmetrical circles of mineral deposits can be seen from the outside. Agate is available in a variety of colors including purple, white, gray, black, brown, red, and pink.

Agate has been used in numerous ancient cultures including the Babylonians,

Egyptians, and some Islamic civilizations too. This stone was used for protection against all kinds of negative energies ranging from falling mildly sick to natural disasters. By anchoring and grounding you firmly to Mother Earth, even today, agate is known for its protective and supportive powers.

This beautiful semi-precious gemstone helps you take things slowly and centers you thereby enhancing your stability and strength. The reason this stone helps you slow down is because its vibrational energy radiates a slow and gentle frequency and soothes you even while relieving stress from your life.

These healing powers can be specifically found in Blue Lace Agate, which is a crystal that is used to calm your troubled mind so that you can articulate your thoughts clearly and confidently. Blue Lace Agate is excellent for balancing and harmonizing the energy frequency of the throat chakra.

By clearing energy blockages in the throat chakra, this crystal improves your communication and listening skills, which is the reason you find yourself being able to speak out honestly and openly without fear and anxiety.

Agate is also great for use if you are struggling to free yourself from a powerful addiction. The grounding power of this stone combined with its ability to soothe and relax you by reducing stress help you overcome addictions. One of the best ways to harness the power of agate is through meditation.

Hold agate crystals in your hand as you meditate and visualize calming light emanating from the stones and firmly grounded you to Mother Earth. Imagine all your problems being absorbed by Mother Earth leaving you feeling stress-free, refreshed, and rejuvenated.

Reach out to the power of an agate crystal during times of crises, changes and transformations or any other difficult periods in your life, and grounded, centered, and protected. There are numerous varieties of agate including but not limited to:

Botswana agate - With a purplish-gray color, Botswana Agate is excellent for smokers who are looking to quit the deadly habit. This particular agate is known to help you focus on solutions rather than on the problems thereby helping smokers and other addicts to overcome their addictions.

Bull's eye agate - This type of agate is also called "Orbicular agate," and is known to ward off evil spirits and curses. It strengthens your fearlessness and helps you survive even in dangerous situations.

Other forms of agate include Brazilian Agate (good for emotional, intellectual, and physical balance), white agate (good for protection of mother and baby during pregnancy), and Blue Lace Agate (already discussed above).

Amethyst

One of the most beautiful and stunning crystals to exist, amethyst has been popular right through the history of humankind. It is found in numerous countries around the world including Bolivia, Brazil, Africa, Mexico, Russia, Canada, the USA, and in Europe too.

Ancient Greeks and Romans used amethyst beads amulets and jewelry. For these ancient civilizations, amethyst was synchronous with luxury, and therefore, this stunning stone was used to adorn crowns, rings, and scepters. Christian bishops wore amethyst rings to symbolize their power and position in the clergy hierarchy.

Also, the purple color of amethyst was the color of royals. The color purple also symbolized allegiance to Christ and to the Christian religion. The Catholic clergymen had amethyst stones on their crosses as the stone is also believed to symbolize celibacy and piety.

The ninth stone on the breast plate (which has 10 stones) of Israel's high priest was amethyst. The ten stones represent the original ten legendary tribes of Israel who took on the voyage to the Promised Land under Joshua after Moses' death, and amethyst represents one of these 10 tribes.

In Greek, the word 'amethyst' translates to 'not drunken.' There is a mythical story behind its name, and it goes something like this. Bacchus, the Greek God of Wine, was once very angry for some reason, and decided to send to send a hoard of ferocious tigers on the first person that tried to cross his path that day. Amethyst, a young Greek virgin, was the unfortunate 'first person' to cross the path of Bacchus. Amethyst was on her way to the Temple of Diana to give thanks to her favorite goddess.

Diana came to the aid of her trusted devotee and before the tigers could attack Amethyst, she was turned into a beautiful, clear crystal. By this time, Bacchus was full of remorse for his reckless and senseless behavior. In an attempt to redeem himself, he poured grape juice over the newly-formed clear crystal rendering the purple color to the stone.

This highly durable and hard stone comes in a variety of purple colors from light lavender to the deep violet shade. Scientifically speaking, the color of the stone is because of the aluminum and iron deposits along with silicon dioxide.

Amethyst is most popularly seen as a protective stone, and is linked to the crown chakra. This purple gemstone is known to purify the mind and help to clear off negative thoughts from it. It also takes care of eliminating stress and anxiety. Meditating with an amethyst crystal is a great way to experience stress relief.

Additionally, amethyst has the power of abundance. So, it relieves stress even while helping you with achieving prosperity. Moreover, amethyst improves your communication and intuitive powers, All these healing properties make amethyst a great crystal to keep in your workplace for added prosperity and career growth, reduced stress and anxiety, and improved leadership skills. When you place an amethyst in your desk at the office, its power will help you make tough decisions based on your gut instinct.

When placed at home, especially in the living room, the amethyst crystal enhances familial bonding and clears the negative energy from the space so that open, fearless conversation can take place between loved ones. Also, place an amethyst in your bathroom and get enhanced relaxation when you take a soothing bath.

Meditate with an amethyst and send up prayers for your life desires and needs to be fulfilled. And watch your prayers being answered by the divine power. Other healing properties of amethyst are:

- It boosts hormone production by tuning the endocrine glands.
- It improves metabolism.
- It has cancer-fighting properties.
- It reduces inflammation and pain.
- It strengthens the immune system.

Amazonite

This green stone is a variety of Feldspar. It is always green in color with cream veins running through the crystal. This soothing stone calms the nervous system including the brain. It also helps t0 maintain optimal physical and mental health.

Interestingly, amazonite also referred to as the Amazon Stone, balances the masculine and feminine energies in your body thereby helping you see both sides of a problem. Consequently, you are able to find innovative solutions for most of your life problems and challenges. It soothes your emotional trauma by reducing fear and worry.

Amazonite helps in healing osteoporosis and other bone-related issues like tooth decay, excessive calcium deposits, and calcium deficiency. It absorbs microwaves and offers protection against electromagnetic radiation.

Aquamarine

Known to be the 19th anniversary stone, aquamarine is great for healing the problems of the throat chakra. Aquamarine is a stone of courage as it soothing and relaxing healing powers calm you down even in the face of challenging adversities. Aquamarine is known as a tranquilizer and helps you move with the flow. If you are a sensitive person, then you will find yourself drawn to this beautiful stone.

In Latin, 'aqua' means water, and 'marine' means 'of the sea.' The name itself is enough to help link this wonderful crystal to the powers of the water kingdom and its myriad healing benefits.

Aquamarine harnesses the soothing power and spirit of the wide, limitless ocean and captures the healing power of life-giving water. Ancient folklore talks about aquamarine as being the treasure of mermaids. Aquamarine helps you reconnect with water, an essential element for the origin of life on this planet.

With powers to improve tolerance and overcome judgmental attitude, the aquamarine crystal offers support to people who feel overwhelmed by huge personal and professional responsibilities. It also sharpens the intellect, clears confusion, and clarifies doubting thoughts and ideas. Also, if you are looking for closure in some long-pending issue in your life, then aquamarine is the stone for you.

From a physical health perspective, aquamarine is excellent for healing sore throats and thyroid related problems. You can meditate with this crystal or wear it as a long necklace around your neck so that all the energy centers in the chest and stomach area can access its healing power.

Like a splash of cold water, aquamarine wakes us from our slothful-like slumbering attitude and urges us to take on life with vim and vigor. It helps us take a break from our boring, habitual routines and reminds us to smell the roses and partake of the beauty of nature that surrounds us.

Aquamarine is also worn before undertaking long voyages for a specific purpose so that you feel fearless and courageous to finish your set task successfully. Wearing aquamarine during such times is like harnessing the power of legendary, fearless seafarers and sailors.

For those people who live close to a water source, aquamarine healing properties work wonders, and for those people who live far away from water, aquamarine connects to the soothing powers of this essential natural element.

Aventurine

Known for its sparkling sheen that glitters when exposed to light, aventurine is a beautiful crystal that gets its particular green color from the mica particular embedded in microcrystalline quartz. India is an important source of green aventurine, the wonderful crystal that is commonly used in jewelry and embedded into boxes or made into little figurines and sculptures. Aventurine is known as the stone of opportunity and can easily form part of your beginner crystal collection, thanks to the economical pricing of the gemstone and its stunning beauty.

Aventurine gets its name from 'Aventura', which is Italian for 'chance or opportunity.' It is believed to be one of the luckiest crystals in the world. In addition to its stunning beauty, aventurine is an excellent remover of negative energies and vibes in your surroundings.

Meditating with aventurine balances and energizes all your chakras and allows for the smooth flow of energy right through your system. It is an excellent de-stressing crystal helping you overcome the frazzled status of your mind and body at the end of a stressful day.

Connecting deeply with the heart chakra, aventurine heals and balances the energy of this crucial energy center allowing you to open your heart to receiving and embracing love from all quarters. It boosts your optimism and fills you with a deep sense of gratitude for everything that life has provided for you.

Black Obsidian

This black beauty is known for protection, growth and self-reflection. The last property listed is the reason for it being known as 'The Mirror.' Black obsidian holds a mirror to you so that you see yourself for who you truly are. As a mirror, this crystal also shows you your inner self. If you find yourself deeply drawn to this stunning crystal, then it could mean that you are in dire need of psychic cleansing.

Black obsidian symbolizes darkness, and it reminds us that we also have dark phases in our life. Black obsidian tells us that instead of running away or hiding from our dark side, we must be strong and brave enough to face it and overcome its bearing on our life. This crystal helps you identify the dark areas in your psyche, which, in turn, helps you clear them away from your life.

In the Paleolithic Age, obsidian was used to make arrows and other tools for daily use by our hunter-gatherer forefathers. Our ancestors also wore it for protection against animal attacks and myriad other dangers that they were exposed to on a daily basis. This stone is also referred to as volcanic glass because it is formed when molten lava cools down quickly. Ancient cultures have also used the power of black obsidian to understand prophecies and other clairvoyant requirements.

Black obsidian works like a psychic vacuum cleaner, and helps you clean up emotional garbage that you might have accumulated over a long period of time. Harnessing the power of black obsidian helps you clear up old and brushed-under-the-carpet emotional debris.

The obsidian stone also protects you from negative emotions like anger, resentment, fear, and different forms of mental, emotional, and physical addictions. Also, the obsidian is great as a stabilizing and grounding crystal and can be most effective to gather scattered energies. Its grounding powers make it most suitable for harmonizing the energies of the root chakra, and one of the most effective ways of harnessing its ability is to place it under your feet while meditating or carrying out healing rituals.

When you feel lost and destabilized, you end up doing all the wrong things in life including putting off important tasks, and also feeling isolated and lonely. During such dark times, black obsidian can be of great use to you. It helps in restoring the balance between your inner self and the physical world, and you see yourself and the world for what they are.

Consequently, your unfocused approach is shed off, and you tend to use your energies in a focused manner resulting in improved outcomes. The obsidian is excellent to keep as a companion during exceptionally long periods of illness and difficulty, especially when handling chronic illnesses. This crystal gives you the strength to overcome obstacles that will keep bombarding you threatening to knock you down. The grounding and stabilizing powers of the obsidian crystal will help you bounce back with added energy. The black obsidian crystal is a truth-enhancing protective stone that protects you and shields you from the harmful effects of negative powers and vibes.

Black Tourmaline

Known for being an excellent energy purifier, black tourmaline protects, secures, and offers stress relief. It acts like a daily disinfectant clearing away negative thoughts and ideas from your mind and keeps your soul free from the harmful effects of these icky thoughts.

You can wear it on a piece of jewelry, keep it in your car, home, or office, or carry it in your pocket. It is a bodyguard stone protecting you from all kinds of negativity. Its ability to absorb electromagnetic radiation makes black tourmaline ideal to place near electronic devices like your PC, laptop, etc.

Place it at the four corners of your home or property and feel its powerful vibration sweeping away all negative energy from your home keeping your loved ones safe and secure.

The 'black' of black tourmaline represents the black shade that has the power to absorb all other frequencies of light. In the same way, black tourmaline absorbs your fears, phobias, anxieties, and other forms of negative thoughts leaving you free to lead a happy, meaningful, and purposeful life.

Tourmaline also comes in a variety of other colors including violet, brown, pink, green, and there is one with a dual pink-green color too. However, black tourmaline is the most commonly occurring color.

Bloodstone

If you have had a bad time in your life recently, then bloodstone is the crystal you have to turn to because it is a powerhouse of rebuilding and restoration. It is a stone, which has the power to restore your disturbed spirit to its original, natural state of joy and bliss.

In Christianity, bloodstone symbolizes Christ's crucifixion. According to legend, when Christ's blood dripped on the earth below his cross, the earth turned to stone, which is referred to as bloodstone. Crystal healers around the world use bloodstone for healing wounds.

This beautiful red stone is great for the root chakra and meditating with it enhances your feeling of safety and security. The properties of bloodstone allows you to see oncoming changes and transformations with a positive perspectives and strengthens your resolve to face them with grit and determination.

Interestingly, the ancient Greeks and Romans were known to wear bloodstone on their body during athletic competitions because this crystal is believed to boost physical strength and endurance. They would dip bloodstone in cold water and then rub it all over their body to promote healing and improve blood circulation. Bloodstone is always believed to work against and protect you from diseases and physical injuries. It was commonly used in European countries before the discovery of penicillin.

On those days when you feel extra tired and sluggish, you can meditate with bloodstone to give you a good kick of energy and get you off your couch-potato attitude. Incidentally, if you find it difficult to sit and meditate using the bloodstone, you can employ the power of walking meditation. Hold the crystal in your hand and practice mindfulness walking to harness the stone's numerous benefits.

Carnelian

With the power to boost your passion, creativity, and confidence, carnelian's powers can invoke the creative child in you. This vibrant, warm stone gets orange-red and brown specks from iron impurities, and the best profile of this crystal is got when it is polished.

The royals from the ancient Egyptian civilizations loved to combine carnelian with Lapis Lazuli and Onyx to create stunning neck pieces in the form of necklaces and collars. This hard crystal was used to rings with carvings and etches of gods and goddesses.

The Viking soldiers wore carnelian to manage stress and anxiety on the battlefield. This sunny vibes of this stunning crystal has the power to bring out the innocent child in you helping you with stress reduction. Carnelian is available in a variety of shades ranging from brown to red to orange.

Carnelian is great to harmonize the energies of the lower three chakras including the root chakra, sacral chakra, and the solar plexus. The fiery spirit of carnelian stimulates the root chakra and circulates vital energy needed to harness your deepest creative instincts and sexual desires.

Whenever you need to display your creative prowess, reach out to the powers of carnelian and access its healing powers. You can keep a small-sized carnelian in your pocket or pouch or wear it as jewelry which can help you access its confidence-building properties right through the day or on special occasions like attending a job interview or an audition, etc.

The healing properties of carnelian include restoring and finding romance and love in your life. It helps you balance the power of love with your sexual drive. Placing carnelian stones over your heart chakra helps you connect with your latent power of passion and romance.

Celestite

This sky-blue crystal connects us with our guardian angels ensuring that we never have to face the storms of life alone. The celestite crystal works like a lullaby as it calms your restless and stormy mind and guides you to love and peace. Just place a small celestite stone under your pillow to ensure a good night's restful sleep and feel rejuvenated to handle the challenges of a new day.

Place the crystal on your third eye chakra and meditate just before you sleep. Not only when your sleep be restful but you will also be able to remember your dreams when you wake, a key element to understand the workings of your subconscious mind.

By restoring your natural inner state of joy, you can achieve calmness and peace if you simply stared into the heavenly blueness of the celestite crystal. Place a stone in your bedroom for tranquility and harmony. Meditate with a carnelian stone in your hand before you go to sleep so that you find the strength and power to overcome the fears and anxieties of nightmares.

The carnelian stone reminds us that beauty of twinkling stars can be experienced only in the absence of sunlight, and therefore, the idea of darkness is not to be feared but to be embraced as another beautiful aspect of nature. Also, it reminds you that no matter how dark things may be, the sun is bound to rise again keeping hopes alive and empowering you to continue your endeavors in your life without fear of failure.

By cooling off your fiery emotions, the carnelian crystals endows you with peace and calmness, which, in turn, clears your mind. Consequently, you find it easy to handle conflicts in your personal as well as professional life. Also, it is a great stone to help you clear your baseless fears about new experiences so that you can try new things in your life, even if these experiences are outside of your comfort zone.

Citrine

With a bright yellow color, the mere sight of this beautiful crystal can light you up. Citrine is like Vitamin C for the soul as it radiates happiness and joy. The name originates from the French word for lime, which is 'citron' and carries a sunny and happy disposition.

The stone is occurs naturally all over the world, including Africa, Brazil, Spain, Madagascar, Scotland, France, Russia, and in many locations across the US. At a cellular level, the atoms of citrine like all other crystals have a repeated pattern which allow crystals to amplify their energy. So, when you fix an intention into you citrine, you can rest assured that the power of your desires will be multiplied and manifested beyond your wildest dreams.

The Ancient Greeks since 300 B.C. have used citrine to adorn and brighten up their jewelry. One of the more modern royalty names that made citrine was Queen Victoria who enhanced the popularity of this magnificent stone by wearing it in the form of jewelry.

Following the fashion trend set up by Queen Victoria in the 17th century, the Scotsmen used citrine as adornments on their sword and dagger handles as well as on their kilts.

Citrine is composed of silicon dioxide, an element that is found naturally in our body, which is the reason why our natural energy resonates with the energy of this crystal. Its unique trigonal shape is also because of the way the energy vibrations affect the molecular structure of the gemstone.

Synchronous with natural autumn colors, citrine symbolizes wealth and abundance. Many crystal healers refer to citrine as 'The Success Stone' or "The Merchant Stone,' thanks to its success-bearing properties that promise wealth, abundance, and growth, especially in your professional and business realms.

Additionally, the energy of this crystal boosts your confidence and motivation driving you to accomplish your goals and achieve success.

Another fortunate feature of citrine is that its energy vibrations can combine that those of other crystals like Garnet or Red Jasper and help to drive your motivation and personal drive. One of the most successful crystals that combine effectively with the power of citrine is clear quartz. This approach will make you work hard which is the most crucial requirement to achieve success.

Citrine has the power to infuse your spirit with positive energy, which is crucial to achieving success and building wealth. The healing effects of the crystal helps to strengthen your mind power to aid in your goal accomplishment process. Connected to the solar plexus chakra, citrine is empowered to strengthen your self-confidence and personal power.

You can place citrine in the following spaces to harness its powerful healing effects:

- Bedroom - for increased abundance and light in your intimately personal life.

- Office space - to enhance creativity and prosperity.

- Children's room - to infuse the environment with positive and cheerful energy.

Wearing citrine jewelry is a great way to keep its power at close proximity at all times. Being in contact with your skin is the perfect way to elevate your sense of optimism, which, in turn, helps you build work hard to progress towards your goals.

Clear Quartz

This stone is the most iconic crystal of the quartz family and is among the most abundantly found minerals across the world, and in almost every continent. This is the reason why clear quartz is spoken of highly and its powers revered in almost every ancient culture of the world.

The word 'quartz' comes from the Greek word for ice because the ancient people believed that it was this crystal is nothing but permanently frozen ice. Here are some of the meanings attributed to clear quartz in the different world cultures:

• In Japan, clear quartz was referred to as the 'perfect jewel' because it symbolizes purity, space, and patience.

• In some of the North American indigenous tribes, clear quartz was seen and worshipped as a sentient being. The stone was giving offerings of food and drink.

• In South American and Australian cultures, clear quartz is an important part of the creation myths. According to the creation myths of both these cultures, the creator of life was a cosmic serpent that was guided by a clear quartz crystal right through the process.

- In South and Central American cultures, it was believed that clear quartz was a vessel or urn that held the spirits of their ancestors. The people of these tribes would carve a human skull with clear quartz and use it as a talisman for funerals and other rituals.

- The natives of Ireland and Scotland carved spheres from clear quartz as talisman. Also, they believed that the powers of clear quartz crystals could keep their cattle safe from diseases and other health problems

Clear quartz is very hard and durable making it highly suitable for a variety of practical purposes. Sand which is nothing but broken down quartz is the essential component of glass, an element used in every nook and corner of the world. The tech industry takes advantage of the programmability of clear quartz and use it in electronic circuits and frequency controls. Moreover, quartz is found in nearly all electronic devices, including mobile phones, LCD TVs, computers, and a lot more.

The programmability and magnifying powers of clear quartz are essential properties for intention manifestations. Clear quartz is a great to program any kind of intentions and you can also delete an old intention and reprogram it with a new one. The crystal's programmable ability in the field of crystals works the same way as in the tech field.

The tricky thing about clear quartz is its ability to magnify any energy found in the surroundings including the negative ones. Therefore, you must remember to cleanse out and recharge your clear quartz crystals regularly and unfailingly.

This beautiful crystal has the power to connect with and heal all the seven primary chakras. However, its energy vibrations are particularly useful to harmonize, balance, and heal the crown chakra. When the crown chakra is at its efficient peak, you can see things clearly and unbiasedly. By clearing the negativities in the crown chakra using clear quartz crystals, you will find yourself being able to eliminate negative perceptions and view everything round in a more objectively and non-judgmentally.

The metaphysical properties of the clear quartz are truly wide-ranging. You can use it to expand your consciousness, stimulate the chakras, and facilitate an environment of openness and honesty. It helps to clear energy blockages in your system to ensure a smooth and unhindered flow of energy right through your body.

Placing a clear quartz crystal near the windowsill will help it radiate and magnify the positive energy from the sun and moon and pass it to the surroundings. You can also transfer your intention into the crystal and meditate with to realize your dreams and desires.

Chrysoprase

If you feel attracted to this stunning green crystal, then it means that you are in need of an emotional makeover. Chrysoprase has the power to spread happiness and optimism in your mind. In fact, in the world of crystals, Chrysoprase is the best known antidepressant. It is an effective prescription for anxiety, depression, and stress as the crystal helps you see things more positively than before.

Closely related to the heart chakra, this crystal's serene and relaxing vibes can help you manage even the most intensely emotional times with ease by soothing and calming your nervous system. Chrysoprase is a great healer of the heart chakra which when energetically well-balanced a smooth flow of positive energy through your heart to the rest of your body. In such conditions, not only is there improved circulation in your physical body but you also feel the power and ability to embrace universal love with increased intensity.

In fact, Chrysoprase which is a variety of Chalcedony (Carnelian being another variety discussed in this chapter) was a favorite gemstone of Alexander the Great. It is believed that he called upon the healing powers of this wondrous crystal before embarking on his voyage of conquering the world.

In ancient times, Chrysoprase was mined and available only in a small place called Lower Silesia near southwestern Poland. The carvings and masonry excavated from Lower Silesia revealed that Chrysoprase was a common crystal used for decorations even as far back as the Iron Age.

The practice of using this variety of Chalcedony in decorative art continued into the 18th century. Frederick II, King of Prussia who conquered this part of Poland got huge amounts of the green rock mined from Lower Silesia and used it to adorn the walls of his palace in Berlin.

The physical profile of Chrysoprase symbolizes a picture of paradise. Just imagine emerald green waters dashing against white sands, and you will see that this picture is exactly what this crystal looks like.

Another crucial element that chrysoprase helps you heal in your mind is to let go of past grudges, forgive, forget, and move on. By activating the heart chakra, this beautiful gemstone allows you to look deep into your mind and get rid of feelings of remorse, regret, revenge, and other negative emotions that you have been bottling up within yourself.

Like jade and rose quartz, chrysoprase is a great healer and harmonizer of the heart chakra helping you not only to get rid of negative emotions that you have been clinging onto for such a long time but also to enhance your power of love and attract universal love in your life.

Conclusion

Crystals can be used in different ways ranging from jewelry to Feng Shui and cleansing chakras. Every crystal has certain inherent properties that help it channel the earth's energy. Each crystal serves a specific purpose, and by learning to use these crystals, you can effectively change the course of your life. Crystal healing is a non-intrusive approach to improve your life! Crystal healing is not a new concept and has been around for a long time. However, it has started gaining popularity as a holistic and alternative approach to healing only in recent times. Learning to heal yourself using crystals is the best way to take charge of your life.

Now that you are armed with all the information you need about crystal healing; it is time to start applying it to your life. Depending on your needs and the areas of your life, you want to work on, use the appropriate crystals. When it comes to crystal healing, you need to be patient and must not stop believing in their powerful energy. You will certainly see a positive change and your overall wellbeing, but it will take some time. So, in the meanwhile, learn to be patient and be consistent while practicing with crystals.

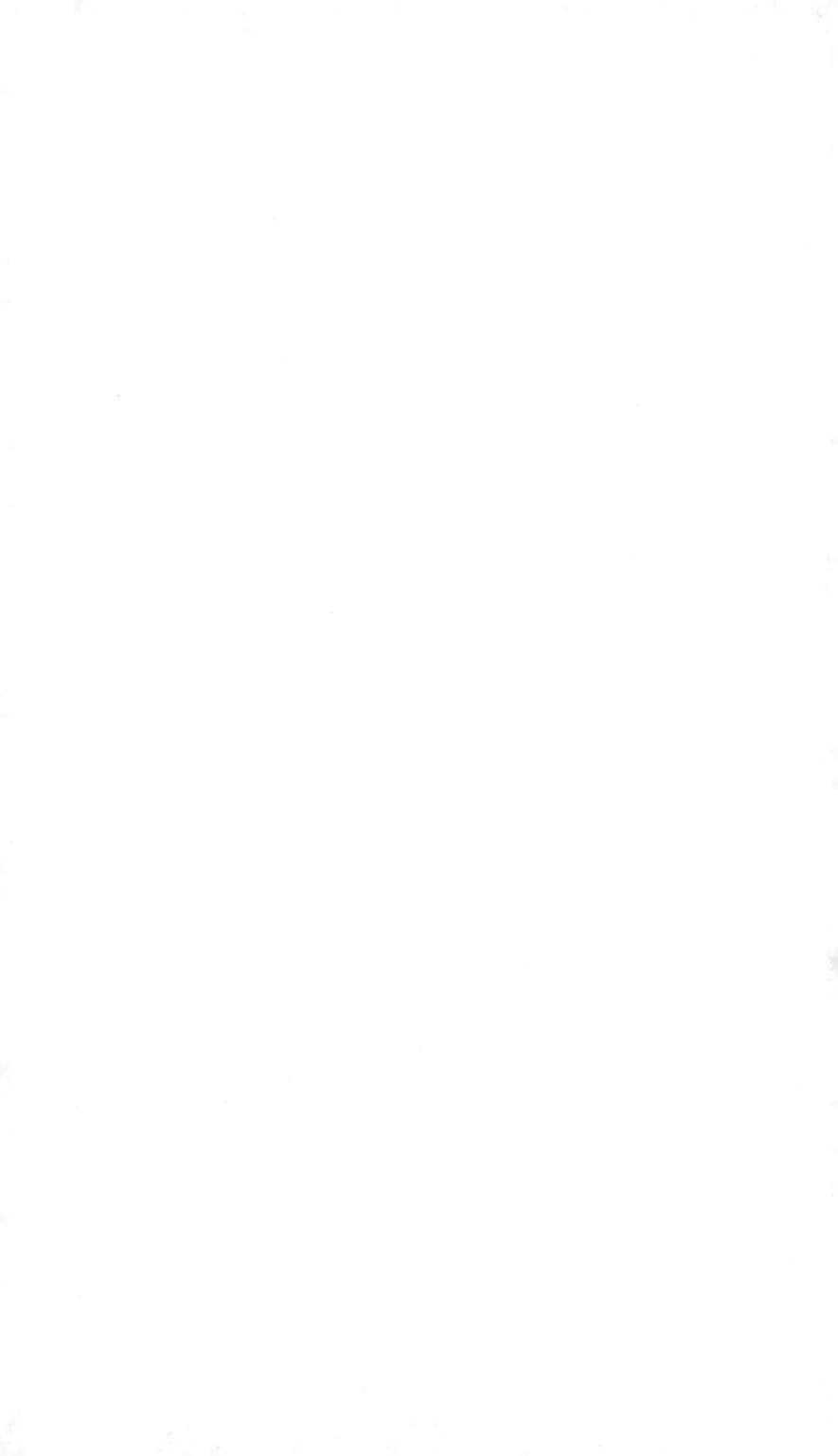